PRAISE FOR *CHIRUNNING*

As yoga teacher in residence and wellness director for the New York Road Runners, I have seen how stiff, tight, and injured runners can become when they think performance is simply about building leg strength and running more miles. Danny Dreyer's insightful approach can change all that. His remarkable program offers a completely new way to run without effort or injury.   **—Beryl Bender Birch, author of *Power Yoga***

I am rarely jolted by today's sports literature, but reading *ChiRunning*, I was thoroughly entranced by the vast wealth of information packed into it. When I realized that on every single page I was making notes of matters crucial to improving my running, I knew I had stumbled upon the most exciting and revolutionary book to hit the running community this decade. It will have you jumping from your seat to discover secrets that will, I believe, perfect and enrich your running experience.

—Toby Tanser, sub-° arathoner,
author of *Train Hard, Win Easy*, cr̶ ̶ ̶mber of
the New York Road Rur̶ ̶tors

As a national-class runner, trained by ̶ ̶ ̶ ̶ coaches, I doubted Danny would have much to ̶ ̶ ̶ know. Fortunately for my teams, as well as my ̶ an open mind. ChiRunning not only helped my level 1, ̶ ̶ ̶ but it improved my running as well! His running technique im̶ ̶performance at all levels and most importantly prevents injuries.

—April Powers, senior head marathon and triathlon coach, team in training, winner Madrid Marathon '83, Olympic Marathon Trials '84, silver medalist Duathlon World Championships, Spain 1997, Wildflower Ironman age group champion '97

The best thing about ChiRunning is that it makes so much sense! The principle of working with your core strength is very powerful and very natural. This program will totally revolutionize the way you run.

—Baron Baptiste, author of *Journey Into Power*

ChiRunning is both spectacularly simple and unique. Danny Dreyer revolutionizes the sport by synthesizing running, tai chi chuan, and applied physics, inventing a new way to run that builds on ancient wisdom. Like the soft and supple power of water to cut through a mountain, he enables runners to propel themselves with less effort, improve their gait, increase their endurance, and knock their socks off by having a really good time.

—Efrem Korngold and Harriet Beinfield, coauthors,
Between Heaven & Earth: A Guide to Chinese Medicine

Danny Dreyer and ChiRunning gave me a precious gift. After being unable to run for ten years because of injury, at age 52 I'm again enjoying pleasurable, injury-free trail runs in the Shawangunk Mountains. I can now move on land with the same economy, flow, and mindfulness that make swimming such bliss for me. I tell people that *ChiRunning* is an owner's manual for anyone who has legs and the desire to use them for health and happiness.

—Terry Laughlin, author, *Total Immersion*

After being unable to run for five years due to a back injury, ChiRunning helped get me back on the road. I highly recommend it for anyone who wants to run without injury.

—Jack Nelligan, M.D., orthopedic surgeon,
former record holder, 400M, Stanford University, Palo Alto, CA

ChiRunning is a great way to practice the principles of Pilates while running. Danny's ChiRunning technique results in fluid movement working from your center. Using only the muscle work you need to be using and letting gravity be your friend lead to efficient movement, one of the key principles of Pilates! ChiRunning and Pilates are totally complementary! I highly recommend Danny's clear explanation of these healthy running concepts. Enjoy in great health.

—Sandra Sweet, owner of Feel Good Fitness,
a Pilates/Movement Education Studio

This book makes running possible for everyone. The magical, concrete guidelines will educate and inspire your every footfall henceforth. Your running will be like play—all energy and no effort. Treat yourself, buy this book NOW and run safely for as long as you like. It's just plain fun to read and the single most useful thing I have ever read about running. Bravo!

—**Jean Couch, director, Balance Center, Palo Alto;**
author of *The Runner's Yoga Book*

Here we have another fine contribution to the awareness of the Tao in sports. This book is in tune with the Taoist wisdom of Wei Wu Wei—Doing Without Doing, to find true joy in the discipline of effortless running as a Way of Being.

—**Chungliang Al Huang, president, Living Tao Foundation,**
coauthor of *Thinking Body, Dancing Mind* **and** *Working Out,*
Working Within, **author of** *Embrace Tiger, Return to Mountain,*
and *Essential Tai Ji*

After 21 years as a sports podiatrist specializing in running injuries and thousands of exams a year, I thought I had seen it all. Then a patient came in who, after taking a ChiRunning class, looked like a different runner—an amazing improvement. It was obvious his impact forces were minimized. Since then I have referred many happy patients to ChiRunning. This technique works to reduce injury, and with it virtually any runner can improve.

—**David R. Hannaford, M.D., podiatrist**

Danny Dreyer has masterfully combined the practice of running with the philosophy of Chi in a beautiful way. People who follow his method will enjoy a more stress-free and graceful way of running and living.

—**Marilyn Tam, author of** *How to Use What You've Got to Get What*
You Want, **and former president of Reebok Apparel & Retail Group**

In our "Learn to Run, Save a Life" training program, ChiRunning has been exceptional. Beginning and experienced runners benefit from the emphasis on injury prevention through efficient biomechanics.

—**Jeff Shapiro, M.D., executive director, Organs 'R' Us;**
race director, Providian Relay (America's second largest relay)

There are many things that distinguish great athletes like Tiger Woods, Barry Bonds or Paula Radcliffe. They have all learned the axiom that less is more. And, they had great mentors. Through this book, Danny Dreyer will become your coach and mentor. He will hand you the keys to a superior running experience. Danny is one of the most generous and talented coaches I know. If you cannot train with him personally, this book is the next best thing.

—**David Deigan, Coach Emeritus,**
San Francisco Road Runners Club; CEO of AFM Inc;
distance runner with over 45 years of experience;
student of ChiRunning

Jerry Fletcher, Ed.D.—Age 61, Corte Madera, CA

I have taken Danny Dreyer's running classes, and they are truly revolutionary. I've been a runner for more than forty years. In my mid-fifties I had knee surgery and was about to give it up. My body just couldn't take the punishment anymore.

Then I took Danny's first workshop (I've subsequently taken advanced ones) and running is a joy again. Despite widespread information in the media about how arthritis in the knees and pain in the lower back is inevitable as we get older, Danny has simply proven them wrong. I'm now running much longer distances than ever (1.5 hours recently), running up steep, long hills, and turning in times on the track that are better than I could do five or ten years ago.

And, more important, it's joyful. I don't end a run in pain. Danny has a concept and a program that can truly revolutionize running.

Darryl Denton—Age 54, San Jose, CA

From the single clinic I did with you I have grown immensely. Through what I learned in your clinic, I am in essence learning to walk again, and learning to run again, and the new ease I am finding there is continuing to spill over into all other aspects of my life.

Mari Anoran—Age 43, Austin, TX

In 1995 I had a serious bicycle accident. I dislocated and broke my ankle in three places and ripped all the major ligaments in my foot. My doctor, who is a top orthopedic surgeon, told me I would never be able to run again. When I took a ChiRunning class I picked up the technique quickly and was amazed that not only could I run again, my performance improved considerably in terms of endurance and ease. I would highly recommend ChiRunning to anyone regardless of age. It's changed my life!

Tim Amyx—Age 44, Mill Valley, CA

After only two sessions with you at the track, I'm completely sold on the ChiRunning style! It has worked wonders for me in the one month I've been applying the techniques to my training and racing. It's amazing! You sold Florencia on it last year, and you've now won me over as well.

Terry Ridgway—Age 36, San Jose, CA

I took your three-session class back in July. After the second session, I ran in the San Francisco Half Marathon and set a personal record by taking nine minutes off my previous best time. Over the rest of the summer I recovered from some minor knee pain and I've been able to stop wearing the knee support straps I'd been using. I then entered the Silicon Valley Marathon. Using the techniques I gained from your class I was able to run the entire race, without taking walking breaks and I completed the distance, taking a whopping 40 minutes off my previous best time!

Patrick Nolan—Age 37, San Jose, CA

I'm amazed and thrilled by your teachings and have already started straightening my spine as I sit and walk. Good Posture is my new mantra.

Cecilia Petersson—Age 36, Hook Norton, England, Women's winner of the 2000 Golden Gate Half Marathon, San Francisco, CA, 2000

I won the women's section in 1:40—and that's thanks to you! It could have been a commercial for the techniques you showed me! Here I was, tiptoeing up that mile-long hill behind other runners who took big strides. And at the crest, I leaned over, got that heel kick going—and gone I was! It was a marvelous feeling! Most of the race felt rather effortless.

Margaret Perrow, Ph.D.—Age 40, Rogue River, OR

Thanks for completely transforming the way I run! What a blast! I really appreciate your sense of humor and enthusiasm, and your understanding that doing things well . . . as well as our bodies allow . . . is *fun!*

Steve Reagan—Age 50, Mountain View, CA

For the last couple of years I have watched my running steadily deteriorate, due to lousy training habits, bad form, various injuries, and over-racing ultras. I must admit that, at first, I was skeptical that anyone could help me overcome my problems but, after only a few months of applying Danny's training methods and using his suggestions for correcting my form, I feel that I am running as well as I ever have over the past several years. I would not hesitate to recommend Danny to anyone who feels that they could use some feedback and coaching to improve their running ability. For once I am looking forward to running an ultra again!

ChiRunning

A REVOLUTIONARY APPROACH TO
EFFORTLESS, INJURY-FREE RUNNING

Danny Dreyer

With Katherine Dreyer

A FIRESIDE BOOK
PUBLISHED BY SIMON & SCHUSTER
NEW YORK LONDON TORONTO SYDNEY

This book is dedicated
to all my Teachers . . . you know who you are.

FIRESIDE
Rockefeller Center
1230 Avenue of the Americas
New York, NY 10020

For information regarding special discounts for bulk purchases,
please contact Simon & Schuster Special Sales at 1-800-456-6798
or business@simonandschuster.com

Designed by Chris Welch
Photography by Lori Cheung © 2003 ThePortraitPhotographer.com

Manufactured in the United States of America

3   5   7   9   10   8   6   4   2

Library of Congress Cataloging-in-Publication Data
Dreyer, Danny.
ChiRunning : a revolutionary approach to effortless,
injury-free running. / Danny Dreyer.
p.   cm.
Includes index.
1. Running—Training.   2. Tai chi.   3. Sports injuries—Prevention.
I. Title: Chi running.   II. Title.
GV1061.5.D74   2004
796.42—dc22   2003065346
ISBN 0-7432-5144-X

Acknowledgments

I would like to pay tribute to the following people for their support in this work. Some have helped me directly and some indirectly, but all have played important roles. I can't imagine playing on a better team.

To Katherine, my partner in every way, thank you for your faith in me and for holding the vision of ChiRunning during my hours of doubt. You remind me that I always have choices, and there is no better gift than that.

Jeff Klein, thank you for your unswerving enthusiasm with this project. Your capacity for seeing the big picture has been immensely reassuring. Bonnie Solow, my angel book agent, your guidance throughout this process has been such a blessing. Caroline Sutton, thanks for all your help and patience in guiding a beginner through a steep learning curve. Lori Cheung, we couldn't have found a more fitting photographer. Your dedication, craftsmanship, and joy have given life to this book. Sonora Beam, thank you for making all of the images possible. Your contribution was giant. A special thanks goes out to Chris, Christina, Marcia, and all you very special folks at Simon & Schuster for enthusiasm and help.

Master Xu, I will be indebted to you forever for teaching me how to bring chi into my life. Your generosity with transmitting ancient Chinese wisdom into the simple act of running fills me with deep respect. Harriet Beinfield and Efrem Korngold, I want to express my thanks for your help and encouragement long before I knew there was a book to be written.

To all the students of ChiRunning, this book is the result of everything you taught me. Thank you also for your feedback, suggestions, and encouragement, which were always timely. Thank you, Jim Dunn, for encouraging me to play along the way. Okay, you can drop the Ox disguise now.

My gratitude goes out to Aga Goodsell, Adriane Steinacker, and Antoinette Addison. You were there at the beginning as students and now you're here in my heart as close friends. Thanks for all those miles together.

Aga, you were the perfect model for the book because the form is so in your body. Thank you for your endless support on many levels.

I am hugely indebted to all of my friends in the ultra-running community. You have been my models for stick-to-it-iveness. And to my larger community of friends and foes, running partners, competitors, and all those who have brought out my best by offering me challenge and support.

I'd like to pay tribute to my wonderful mother, my first teacher, and the one who has had to put up with me for more years than anyone else.

And finally to my daughter, Journey. You are the inspiration behind all that I do. May you grow up with a generation of peers that looks to the heavens for knowledge and listens to their bodies for the Truth.

Contents

Running Lessons
from a T'ai Chi Master

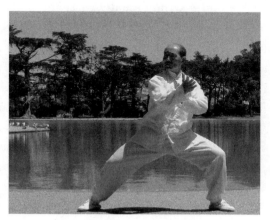

Master George Xu

Not long ago, I was running past a grade school. It was a warm, late-spring day, and the kids were out on recess. They were busy playing tag and chasing balls and just doing what kids do best—running around. I stopped to take a swig of water from my bottle, and as I watched the flurry of little legs, I was reminded once again why I love to watch kids run. Every one of them had perfect running form: a nice lean, a great stride opening up behind them, heels high in the air, relaxed arm swing and shoulders. They had it all! One of my biggest desires as a coach is to help adults learn to run like they did as kids. It's such a natural movement when kids do it. It looks so effortless and joyful. Many books about running tell you to just go out and run like you did as a kid. There's just one problem with that suggestion: You don't have the same body today that you did back then. If you do, I'd like you to be my teacher.

So why don't adults run like kids, with that same ease and joyful-ness? After running for thirty years and working with thousands of runners, I'd have to say that the two biggest factors are stress and ten-sion. I can speak for myself, and maybe you can relate. Since I left the sixth grade, I have put my body through a wide range of physical and emotional stresses, such as tightening my shoulders when I'm wor-ried, slouching all day at my desk, holding tension in my neck while driving—the list is endless. Individually, these might not sound like a big deal, but when you add them all up over a lifetime, they have a major cumulative effect on how you move. I've also done a few radical things that have taken a bit more of a toll on my body, like skiing off cliffs and doing face plants while skateboarding. As Carolyn Myss, author of *Anatomy of the Spirit,* would say, "Your biography becomes your biology." With all of this abuse stored in my body, I'd be hard-pressed to run like I did as a kid. The good news is that for anyone with a little patience and perseverance, it is possible to get back to that state.

There are over 24 million runners in the United States alone. But get this. It is estimated that 65% of all runners incur at least one in-jury a year that interrupts their training. That means that 15.6 mil-lion people will get injured this year from running. No wonder people have a love/hate relationship with running. It's one of the most ac-cessible and inexpensive ways to stay in shape, yet it poses a danger that is cautioned in articles, books, and doctors' offices everywhere. Most people treat injury as part of the sport and learn to accept that it will happen sooner or later: "I'll deal with it when it happens." It's the same line I get when I ask people in the San Francisco Bay area if they worry about earthquakes.

The conclusion I've come to after teaching countless runners is that *running does not hurt your body.* Let me repeat that—and you can read my lips—*running does not hurt your body.* It's the *way* you run that does the damage and causes pain.

When Adriane, 42, came to me, she was caught in a back-and-forth cycle of training hard to get into good condition, then getting injured and having to lay off for a couple of weeks, then starting all over again. She thought it was the right thing to constantly train fast and strength-train to improve her times in the marathon. But she was not making any forward progress because of the nagging injuries and her own internal pressure to keep increasing her weekly race-training schedule. With the ChiRunning technique, she learned how to relax while running and, more important, in the other areas of her life. She realized that she was not only a driven runner, she was a driven person. Without all the tension in her body, she stopped injuring herself while running, and her training took on a new level of consistency.

Jerry, a 59-year-old runner, was just about to give up running when he came to his first ChiRunning class. He had been a runner for forty years, and after having knee surgery, he had begun to feel the same old aches and pains creeping into his runs that had prompted the surgery. He was afraid that if he continued running, he would ruin his knees and live in pain for the rest of his life. It has now been two years since his first class, and he is running regularly—including an hour and a half on steep trails once a week—and looking forward to many more years of pleasurable running. In fact, he wrote to me recently, thrilled that he had finished first in his age group in a local race, something he had never dreamed of even before his surgery.

Carmen, 35, was a beginning runner and insecure about her ability to do anything well physically. After taking a series of three ChiRunning classes, she happened to call as my wife, Katherine, and I were reviewing her class on video. Katherine remarked on how good Carmen looked in the film and asked her how she liked the class. "Oh, it simply changed my life" was the reply. "For the first time in my life, I feel like I can be good at a sport."

From beginners to competitors to the forty-plus crowd who are afraid of injuring themselves as they get older, ChiRunning is meeting the needs of runners with an approach that builds a healthy body instead of breaking it down from misuse or overuse.

ChiRunning Versus Power Running

The current paradigm of running form and injury prevention is founded in muscle strength. It is basically built around three principles: (1) If you want to run faster, you need to build stronger leg muscles. (2) If you want to run longer, you need to build stronger leg muscles. (3) If you want to avoid or recover from injuries, you need to build stronger leg muscles. Do you see a theme developing here? It's all dependent on muscles to get the job done, and the leg muscles are given the bulk of the responsibility to make it all happen. That's a lot of responsibility and, according to T'ai Chi principles, a very unbalanced way to move your body. The problem with strength training is that it doesn't get to the root of the most common cause of injury: poor running form. Most runners want to run either longer or faster at some point in their running career, but without good running form, added distance will only lengthen the time you are running improperly and increase your odds of getting hurt. If you try to add speed with improper running form, you are magnifying the poor biomechanical habits that could cause injury. So, the best place to build a good foundation is in getting your running motion smooth, relaxed, and efficient. Then you can add distance or speed without risking injury.

This book presents an alternative to what we call power running. ChiRunning is based on the centuries-old principle from T'ai Chi that states, *Less is more*. Getting back to that childhood way of running doesn't come from building bigger muscles, it comes from relaxing muscles, opening tight joints, and using gravity to do the work instead of pushing and forcing your body to move in ways that can do it harm. Most runners, especially those over 35, will tell you that running can keep you in good shape but it's hard on your body. I developed ChiRunning because I really didn't believe that pounding and injury should be a part of running. I just didn't buy it.

I've never considered myself a great runner. I liked to run as a kid, but I shied away from it in high school because, to tell you the truth, I was intimidated by the caliber of our track-team members, most of whom could run a hundred-yard dash in under 10 seconds and a quarter mile in under a minute. In an inner-city high school with 3,600 students, the coaches could basically pick from the cream of the crop, and I hardly considered myself even potential cream. So I joined the ski club and partied instead. In fact, I signed up to take gymnastics, because every Wednesday the gym classes had to run around a nearby lake, and I couldn't imagine making myself run for twelve minutes without stopping.

Don't get me wrong. I've always loved sports, and I love to learn new things with my body. Whenever I wanted to take on a new sport, I would apply another love of mine—figuring out how things work. As far back as I can remember, I've always had questions running through my mind, like: "Why does a clock tick?" or "What kind of machine wraps a stick of butter?" As a kid, I loved taking things apart to see what made them do what they did, then I'd try to put them back together again. Although I had a lifetime average of about 75% on the reassembly, I always figured out how they worked.

This is what I did with skiing, rock climbing, and sailing. I broke each sport down into its elemental parts, which would then give me a physical understanding of how to put it all together into a unified movement. As I found myself improving, I would get more excited and consequentially focus even more. My learning was driven by my passion, so my hours spent practicing would fly by. I loved learning new body skills.

In my early twenties, when I took up running, I approached it in much the same way. I began running regularly in 1971, when I got drafted into the army. Running around the army base at an easy pace was very relaxing for my body and helped to settle my mind. This was the first time I had used a sport for more than physical fitness: I wasn't into being in the army, so I used running to escape the barracks and explore. After doing an eighteen-week stint with Uncle Sam, I was graciously given an honorable discharge, but not before discovering a new favorite pastime.

When I was a young adult, my curiosity about how things worked extended into those unseen forces out of which the physical world springs forth. I was no longer satisfied with only understanding the *how*, I wanted to know *why* they worked. I always came away with a sense that there was more going on than I was seeing. For lack of a better term, I call it the invisible world, and my curiosity about it is still the driving force behind my approach to life. It eventually led me to the study of T'ai Chi and using chi in my running.

The same year I started running, I began my investigation of the invisible by practicing long hours of meditation with a teacher from India. The most important knowledge I gained was how to quiet my mind so I could listen to my body. As my meditation practice began to spill into my running, my running became more and more an exploration of my own physical nature and the energies powering it.

Fast-forward to 1991. Over a period of twenty years, my running and my exploration of the invisible had become increasingly intertwined. I began running longer and longer distances as a means of exploring the potential of my body, which is what led me to the sport of ultramarathon running (distances longer than 26.2 miles). In 1995 I ran my first race, a fifty-miler in Boulder, Colorado. Since then I have completed thirty-four ultramarathons, winning my age group in fourteen of them and placing in the top three in my age group in all but one. The distances I have raced are 50K (31 miles), 50 miles, 100K (62 miles), and 100 miles. In 2002 I ran my first marathon (the Big Sur International Marathon), winning my age group in a time of 3:04, which I was very pleased with, considering there's about a thousand feet of vertical gain on the course.

Now, I just have to say right here, the ChiRunning technique is *not* about running super-long distances. I have chosen ultradistance running as a way to learn about my body, but I don't necessarily recommend it for everyone. If you are so inclined, ChiRunning certainly makes distance running more enjoyable, but even more important, it represents a way to move your body by using mental focus and relaxation instead of muscle power. In this book you will learn about the principle of "Form, Distance, and Speed," which means that you start by building a foundation of correct running form. As your foundation gets stronger, your body will be able to handle more distance. Then speed becomes a by-product of good technique practiced over increased distance, not something dependent on the size and strength of your muscles. Ultimately, you're not working to build distance and speed, you're working to build *presence,* and that can happen at any distance or speed.

When I first started running ultras, they were hard work. Along the way I had bouts with aches and pains, which I tried to approach with a positive attitude, telling myself, "If you can get this right, you might not have this pain again." At one point in my training, I had a knee pain that would start about twenty miles into my long run. But I never blamed the running for injuring my body. Instead, I took full responsibility by always trying to figure out how my form was causing my knees to hurt. I assumed that it was a matter of making the right correction, and I let that premise guide me in my trial-and-error research.

In 1997 my eyes were opened to a whole new realm when I met Zhu Xilin, a T'ai Chi master from China who introduced me to the concept of moving from one's center and letting the arms and legs follow. His way of moving his body looked both effortless and powerful. Needless to say, adapting this idea to my running was a huge draw for me.

T'ai Chi owes its origins to the study of animal movements. According to the Chinese, chi (pronounced *chee*) is the energy force that animates all things. It runs through a system of meridians that distribute this energy to all parts of your body. By practicing mental focus and relaxation, one can learn to sense and direct this subtle energy through the system of movements and exercises known as T'ai Chi. This concept is downplayed by Western medicine because chi cannot be detected with measuring instruments and cannot be supported by the scientific method. The interesting part about chi is that it will move through your body whether you believe in it or not, because if it weren't running through you, you'd be dead. Fair enough?

The current trend in sports training toward using one's core muscles is just starting to scratch the surface of knowledge the Chinese have been developing for three thousand years. One of the things T'ai Chi teaches us is to direct movement from points along our spine; thus it can originate from the center line of your body and not from the peripheral. Observation of Nature teaches us that the strength of a tree lies in its trunk, not in the branches and leaves. Why should the human body be any different? Why do you think the area of your body that houses all your vital organs is called your trunk? Are we nodding yet?

Look at the movement of a cheetah, the fastest land animal on earth. It doesn't have big strong legs like a tiger. It has skinny legs like a greyhound. So how does it go so fast? The secret lies in its spine, which is where most of its chi energy is contained. When a cheetah runs, you can see that its source of power comes from the spine and not the legs.

For your legs to be powered by the chi energy coming through the spine, they need to be very relaxed. Master Zhu would constantly tell me to keep my spine straight but relax the rest of my body and let the chi flow through "like water through a pipe." A major lightbulb went off in my head when it occurred to me that this idea could be applied to running.

I started to grasp the idea of moving my body from its center and letting my legs be pulled along for the ride. But relaxing my arms and legs while running only uncovered the next problem in the chain— the need to relax my shoulders and hips. Once I became adept at relaxing, I could feel how much power my spine had when it wasn't met with any resistance from the rest of my body. That was when I began to experience a new level of smoothness and ease, often feeling as if I were skimming along on a conveyor belt. As I worked on technique, my sense of running more smoothly and efficiently gradually began to replace that old feeling of working hard to run. My breathing became less labored, my muscles were not getting sore, and many times I would feel better at the end of a run than I did when I started. I could go out for a thirty-mile run and come back without any major discomfort: an exhilarating realization. "Postrun recovery" began to take on a whole new meaning—hours instead of days, and sometimes no time at all. This is when I realized that I was onto something *very* cool. Since my discovery in 1998, I have not had a running injury of any kind (knock on wood), despite a heavy teaching, training, and racing schedule.

In 1999 I moved from Boulder to San Francisco, feeling a great sense of loss at having to leave Master Zhu. When I first arrived, I ran through Golden Gate Park, looking for a new T'ai Chi teacher. Each day I'd see many small groups practicing their moves, and there would be Master Xu, who always had only one student. He would be manually moving his subject into various postures, like an artist shaping a clay figure. He was totally attentive to his students in a way that

I never witnessed in any of the other teachers. After seeing him numerous times at the same spot, I decided to ask him if he would be my teacher. I introduced myself and said, "I don't care if I ever learn T'ai Chi, but I want to learn how to apply what *you* do to my running." His face lit up. "I've always had a theory," he said, "that one could take all the principles of T'ai Chi and use them in any sport. Come back in three months."

That was it. He never gave me his name or phone number. Just "Come back in three months." What could I say? So, after ninety days of waiting, I went back and found him in the same spot where I left him. I reminded him who I was, to which he responded, "Okay, start tomorrow." I fully expected him to end his sentence with "grasshopper." As it turns out, George Xu is an internationally known T'ai Chi master who leads seminars all over the world and has produced an extensive collection of videotapes documenting many Chinese masters of almost every martial art in China. Since that day, Master Xu (pronounced "shoe") has had a huge impact on the further development of what I have come to call ChiRunning. He has not only confirmed and clarified all that I'd discovered prior to meeting him, he has helped me to synthesize the themes of T'ai Chi with what I've learned about running.

I've always loved to watch people run. It's wonderful to see how many different types of bodies there are and how many different ways they run. But if you want to see what's really going on with a runner, watch her face. If you watch children run, they're generally all smiles. But what I see more often than not in adults is an expression that ranges somewhere between discomfort and terror. Lots of folks leave me with the impression that they're not enjoying themselves. No wonder running has a bad rap. What happened to all those smiles?

We need to reeducate ourselves to move in the ways we were designed to move. Most people are never taught how to run. It's one of those things we all take for granted because everyone runs soon after learning to walk. Go to any fitness center or gym or continuing-education catalog, and you'll find classes in every sport on the planet *except* running. This was a big part of what convinced me to become a full-time coach and running instructor. As I brought more of the inner focuses of T'ai Chi into my running classes, the students began to see immediate and dramatic changes in their performance and outlook. Since introducing the ChiRunning technique to the general public, I've seen many of those smiles reappear.

Through my T'ai Chi teachers, I have learned that losing the beautiful ease of movement we had as children is part of the process of maturing as a human being. Children move naturally but not consciously. It is our job, as adults, to learn how to consciously move through life with that same flow and beauty. It is through conscious action and understanding that we can become masters of our bodies and ourselves. The ChiRunning technique is the vehicle that will allow you to experience once again what it's like to run with a sense of power and connection in your body.

I still don't consider myself an exceptional runner. When I run, I rely almost entirely on inner focuses and technique rather than on talent or physical strength. Ultimately, ChiRunning is not about being an accomplished runner, it's about what you come away with. It's learning how to listen to your body and adjust appropriately to improve your form and enhance your performance. It's learning how to sense your body, your actions, and the results of your actions; how to learn from what you do and what you feel. It's learning how to use running as a vehicle to discover yourself on many levels.

If you would like to improve your running form, have fewer injuries, develop your own training program, and be able to run into your old age, then this book is for you.

If you would like to increase your overall health and well-being, this book is for you, too.

If you would like to learn to be more centered and have more of a mindful approach to your running and your life, this book is also for you. ChiRunning is not so much about the running as it is about the chi. It's about having a focused and energetic relationship with your body. It means learning how to be your own best friend, teacher and guide—how to be mindful, quiet, and energetic all at the same time. Sound great? It is.

How to Use This Book

I'd like to take a minute here and clue you in on what to expect in the coming chapters. As a fair warning, I do not get into explaining the technique of ChiRunning until Chapter 4. So if it feels like I'm taking forever to get to the good stuff, there's a reason. This book tells you not only how to be a better runner, it also offers you the opportunity to develop qualities from running that you can use in the rest of your life. This approach to running is best understood when you can see the background and logic supporting it. The first three chapters are dedicated to laying out the philosophical foundation, so when I give you the specifics of the technique, they will all make sense.

Chapter 1 compares the present paradigm of running, power running, to ChiRunning, the proverbial new kid on the block.

Chapter 2 introduces you to the five *Principles*, or natural laws, upon which T'ai Chi and ChiRunning are based. When your movements are in sync with the laws of Nature, you have one of the best support systems around, to put it mildly.

Chapter 3 will explain to you the "inner" skills of ChiRunning, which I call *Chi-Skills*. Learning these four mind/body skills will change your running into an entirely new activity.

Chapter 4 introduces you to the ChiRunning *focuses*, which are the specific physical and mental methods used to run more smoothly, efficiently, and injury-free.

Chapters 5 through 9 teach you how to bring the ChiRunning technique into your running program including program development, peak performance training, and diet. Chapter 10 then tells you how to bring the ChiRunning principles into your everyday life.

I would suggest reading the book straight through once. Then go back and reread portions that you didn't feel clear on. My favorite trick with a manual is to mark all of my favorite sections with a tab, labeled for easy reference. If you want something more permanent and reliable, go to your local office-supply store, buy some stick-on plastic tabs, and go crazy. I'd mark all the exercises, drills, focuses, and tips so you can access the information easily if you're on your way out the door for a run. Believe me, you will use this book more often if you have a system in which the information is at your fingertips.

I've found that the body and mind learn best through repetition. For this reason, I recommend that you reread this book several times, then at least once a year, to keep your mind and body refreshed with the process and terminology. Take your time, and you'll learn more, faster.

Learning the basic ChiRunning technique can take anywhere from one to three months for the average runner, but the greater knowledge gained from the approach will be something that, when practiced regularly, will influence your thoughts and actions for the rest of your life.

CHAPTER ONE

ChiRunning: A Revolution in Running

A good runner leaves no footprints.—Lao Tzu, Tao Te Ching

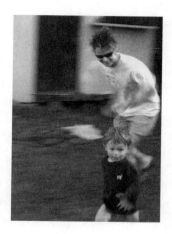

A s Emily ran past our group at the track, we all remarked at what beautiful running form she had. She seemed to float across the ground so effortlessly that you could hardly hear her feet touch down. The moment seemed almost otherworldly, and she became the role model for everyone in the class.

Emily is a 3-year-old whose parents were taking a ChiRunning class at the track that day.

Children run naturally. When they want to catch their friends in a game of tag, all they do is focus on who's It, and their body just follows along. They're not thinking about running. They're enjoying the game of tag and having so much fun running that there is very little work going on. Since little effort is involved in their movement, there is little chance for injury. There isn't any pounding in their joints or any tension in their muscles that could be the hot spots for pain to reside. How could there be, when their movement is based on fun and play?

Sarah Hughes, upon winning the gold medal in women's figure skating at the 2002 Olympics, said, "I wasn't thinking of a gold medal, I went out to have fun and a great time. . . . All I wanted to do was skate my best." It was easy to see how much fun she was having. Her sense of freedom and joy allowed the energy in her body to fill the arena, infectiously sparking the audience. On the other hand, Michelle Kwan, five-time world champion, was caught by the camera just as she was about to go on the ice. The anxiety in her face displayed the pressure she was under to produce a gold medal for her country. She looked anything but relaxed and playful. My heart went out to her. The tension that she was carrying prevented her best energy from moving through her body, resulting in a performance below what she was capable of and landing her the bronze medal.

I would venture to say that most of us could run pretty easily back when we were in grade school and not feeling pressured to perform. But we have since lost that wonderful sense of ease. Like Michelle, we often have performance anxiety that makes us uptight and blocks us from feeling ourselves and doing our best. In order to regain this ease and joy, we need to consciously teach our bodies how to relax and move so that running can feel as effortless as it once did.

A great way for me to learn to relax has been my study of perceived effort level (PEL). Your PEL is the amount of exertion you sense from yourself. Let's say that Joan is an average runner in decent shape. She goes out for her morning run and puts in a few miles at a 9-minute-per-mile pace. She's been doing it for weeks, and she has a distinct physical sensation of what that pace feels like. To her it feels like a nice, comfortable, easy pace. Then she goes to a party that evening and dances to some great rock and roll after having a couple of beers. The next morning she drags herself out of bed to run with her next-door neighbor, who also likes to run at a 9-minute pace. As they get into their run, she asks him how fast they're going, because it feels like a bit much. He tells her that they're exactly on pace: 9-minute miles on the button. Meanwhile, she's feeling like she's hustling to catch a crosstown bus. Her legs are tired, she's breathing like a freight train, and she's not sure how much longer she can keep it up. Her PEL feels *way* higher than it was yesterday, though they're running the very same pace.

Perceived effort is what you *feel* like you're doing, regardless of what you are *actually* doing. The emphasis of ChiRunning is to set yourself up so there are no energy blocks in your body. This means three things: maintaining good posture; keeping your joints open and loose; and making sure your muscles are relaxed and not holding any tension. If you're practicing these, your PEL will feel lower than it normally does, at whatever speed you are capable of sustaining. As your running form becomes increasingly efficient, you will be able to run faster and/or longer at a lower PEL. There's no reason why getting into great shape needs to hurt or feel strenuous, and there's no reason on earth why it can't be fun. As your ability to run well increases, so will your sense of joy. Likewise, as your joy increases, so does your ability to run well.

The ChiRunning technique will completely alter the way you approach running, because it combines relaxation with biomechanically correct running form. This book is designed to train your mind to focus and direct your movements so your body doesn't have to work as hard. One of my favorite quotes from Master Xu is "The body wears out . . . the mind lasts forever."

A Sampling

Here's a sample exercise that will give you a sense of PEL. It will help you feel the difference between using lots of leg muscles to move your legs (hard work/higher PEL) and using your core muscles (easy work/lower PEL).

- Set this book down and stand up straight and tall.
- Walk in place for 10 seconds, picking up your feet.
- After walking in place for 10 seconds, bend over at the waist—like you're bowing—and walk in place for another 10 seconds.
- Now straighten your body to the vertical position and keep walking in place for a few seconds.

How did it feel to "walk" bent over? How did it feel when you straightened up your body? Was it any easier?

Here's what's happening. When you stand tall and upright, your psoas muscle (pronounced "so as") is stretched, and it acts somewhat like a rubber band to lift your leg when you walk in place. Those psoas muscles are some of the strongest core muscles in your body, working to lift the weight of your feet, which means there's a *large* muscle group doing a *tiny* job. That's why your PEL is lower.

When you bend at the waist, your psoas is collapsed, and you have to lift the weight of your leg with your quadriceps, which feels like more work. As you straighten up, your psoas is engaged, and the work of lifting your legs feels easy again. In this exercise, you should sense a lower PEL when you're standing upright, lifting your legs, than when you're bent over. If you sense that standing tall while picking up your feet is the easier way to go, that's because it is. This exercise is intended to give you a sense of how much harder your legs have to work when you're not holding your posture in a straight line. In Chapter 4 I will talk about how to take your nice, straight posture and tilt it forward to lower your PEL while running.

Before I get into telling you more about how running will be easier, let's talk about why you would want to run at all.

THE BENEFITS OF RUNNING

Let's put it this way: I might sound like a fanatic, but I love running. It's like having an old friend that is always there when I need a lift in spirits. Once I get myself out the door, the world opens up, no matter how hemmed in or bummed out I might be feeling. I can call a friend to come along and explore a new trail or spend a morning cruising canyons and watching waterfalls. Running gets you outside, and if you run all year long, it does a wonderful job of keeping you in touch with the changes of the seasons.

You know what else happens while I'm out there having the time of my life? My heart gets stronger, my bone density increases, I burn a ton of calories, and my aerobic capacity improves. Not bad for a day of play.

It's inexpensive and requires minimal gear. You can run almost anytime and anywhere. And there is nothing like a good run to clear your mind and put life's problems into a more sane perspective. When you travel to a new city, it's a great way to learn the lay of the land and get an intimate feel for your new surroundings. One of my favorites; it's a great way to cleanse my body of overindulgences.

You can also develop qualities from running that can be transferred into the rest of your life, like perseverance or consistency or will-power. Maintaining a solid running program teaches you how to set goals and work toward them, how to develop a strategic action plan, and how to use setbacks as lessons. In fact, there is almost no situation in your life that cannot be approached and handled from what you learn about yourself through running. Running can be a study of life itself.

WHY PEOPLE GET INJURED

For all the good that can be gained from running, it is also fraught with many potential dangers to your body. It can damage your knees, shins, hips, and back. It can take its toll on your feet, and it has even been said to damage your eyesight (from all the jarring and pounding). People are led to believe that running inherently creates these injuries. That's a myth I would like to put to sleep.

I believe the primary causes of injuries are poor running form and poor biomechanics. Running is a natural movement. Poor biomechanics cause you to move your body in an unnatural way, which leads to undue stress on muscles, joints, and ligaments; these areas then become vulnerable to injury. The most common theory says the primary cause of running injuries is overtraining. I believe this to be a myth as well, although it is a factor, especially in result-oriented training. If you have poor running form, you can injure yourself at any distance. I've seen people get shin splints after half a mile. When there is an imperfection in your biomechanics, it will eventually show up as an ache or pain. You need only run far enough, and each of those little imperfections will eventually take its toll on your body. I guarantee it.

The upside is, by improving your biomechanics and your running form, you greatly decrease your odds of getting injured at *any* distance or speed.

Paul, age 35, was an average runner who wanted to challenge himself to complete a marathon. The farthest he had ever gone was six miles, because every time he ran, his shins would start hurting in the first mile, to the point where they hobbled him. He came to a ChiRunning class in July, with a goal of running the Honolulu Marathon in early December. With the help of the ChiRunning technique, he was able to run all of his mileage upgrades while decreasing the pain level in his shins. After months of dedicating himself to his new running form, he was able to run his first marathon in 3:37 without the debilitating pain of shin splints. He told me later that he would not have thought it possible to complete a marathon before working on his form. Now he's thinking of trying to qualify for the Boston Marathon!

I would attribute almost all injuries to the current paradigm of running, which I call power running.

POWER RUNNING: NO PAIN, NO GAIN

No doubt about it, that macho catchphrase is still getting airtime, like it's some kind of badge of honor. It doesn't matter whether you're talking about running programs, international relations, or making a pie crust, there are better ways to move through a project than by force.

Power running can best be explained from two angles: technique and mind-set. Both the technique and mind-set of power running are reflected in the "no pain, no gain" attitude that pervades Western sports and thinking. Don't get me wrong. Power running does work, but at quite a cost. I just keep thinking about those fifteen plus million runners who are getting injured *each year*, and I know this doesn't have to be the case.

THE METHOD

The predominant theme of power running is to develop leg strength and leg speed to run faster and farther. Power running also emphasizes regular training to get your legs stronger, which will help you run better and avoid injuries.

From a training standpoint, building and using more muscles are hard work for the body and even more difficult for us folks over fifty. Any increase in muscle usage requires more time on strength training and creates a greater propensity for injury. Then more fuel is required to power these muscles; more metabolic waste (lactic acid) is produced; and more time is needed for recovery after running, especially after races or hard workouts. It makes me tired and achy just thinking about it.

There are many exercise plans designed to build stronger calves, quads, and buns of steel so that you can become a better runner. A significant amount of training time is encouraged to improve one's leg strength and thereby performance.

I recently read about a comparative study in Denmark of the difference between Danish runners and Kenyan runners. Here's what they had to say, according to a recent article in the *Kamalpa Monitor:*

> In all, it was discovered that Kalenjin [Kenyan] elite runners as well as Kalenjin untrained boys have a superior running economy compared to their Danish counterparts probably due to the fact that the Kalenjins have more slender legs and thus use relatively less energy when running.

Well, they got part of it right. The Kenyans are using relatively less energy, but it's not because their legs are skinny. It's really the other way around: Their legs are slender *because* they have such excellent running economy. They're so efficient that they don't need big muscles. The Kenyans are winning everything from 10Ks to marathons with those "slender legs." Yet, according to the power-running paradigm, it takes strong leg muscles to run fast. Something isn't adding up here. I'd say what's winning races is their technique, which shares many of the characteristics of ChiRunning—two examples being their lean and foot strike. The Kenyans have a beautiful forward lean when they run, which does two things: It allows gravity to assist in pulling their body forward, and it allows them to land on their midfoot instead of their heels, thus avoiding the braking motion of the heel strike, which is common in most other runners.

Power running can be detrimental to runners because it does not address the real cause of most injuries, which is poor biomechanics. Instead, it focuses almost entirely on building stronger muscles as a solution for recovering from or avoiding injuries. It's true, strengthening muscles will buy you some time. But until you correct the real cause of the injury, odds are you're going to get the same injury again.

For instance, if you have shin splints, you can take time off to heal and then strengthen the anterior tibialis (shin muscle) by walking on your heels. But if you're using the same running form that created the shin splints, that muscle will eventually tire, and you'll get them again. With the ChiRunning technique, you won't be pushing off with your toes (the primary cause of shin splints), and you'll barely use your shin muscles. Shin splints will become a nonissue, and you won't have to build and maintain stronger muscles to compensate for your running form.

THE POWER-RUNNING MIND-SET

The mind-set of power running is result-oriented, which I feel is the primary cause of overtraining. Thus, people can get an idea about how fast or far they should run that is not necessarily based on a reality in their body.

This is not only a setup for disappointment, it's a recipe for injury. Overtraining can be defined as training beyond the level at which your body is currently capable. If you're a beginning runner and you're following a training book that says you should be running 2 miles, 3 days a week, you could be a candidate for overtraining. What if you've never run a mile?

If you're driven to do more than you're capable of, you are usually driven by something *external.* It could be a desire triggered by an inspirational article in a running magazine, or an impulse you get from watching a great athlete on TV. Here are some external motivators to beware of:

- Wanting to do better because of peer pressure
- Trying to match the speed of your running partners
- Wishing to be faster than you were last year
- Needing to prove your value to your parents
- Wanting to keep up with your significant other
- Being anxious to lose those last fifteen pounds before your wedding day
- Hoping to run a marathon by a certain age or date
- Needing to run faster to keep up with your dog

The list is endless, and in case you didn't notice, they're *all* products of a result-oriented mind-set.

There are plenty of external ideas to be motivated by, but the motivators that really get things rolling and generate successes are the ones that come from the *inside*. Unfortunately, our Western culture is increasingly shaped by the world of marketing, which has at its root the mission to pull you off center and outside of yourself so you'll buy whatever product or service is put before you. A lot of power running buys into the images that we are constantly bombarded with, like "bigger is better" or "survival of the fittest" or everybody's favorite, "No pain, no gain." Just look at the covers of any current running or fitness magazine, and you'll be hit with alluring catchphrases like: "You too can have rock-hard abs!" or "Have a hard body in six days!" Right, but what about those of us who are over 18?

Almost everyone I see is power running (except the Kenyans), and for decades it has been the approach used by every level of running coach from middle school through college. But when I think of that statistic of a 65% yearly injury rate for running, combined with the incredible success rate of the Kenyans, I can't help but believe that there is something seriously wrong with the way we're approaching the sport. We need a paradigm shift, away from the power-running approach, and ChiRunning represents that shift.

THE "CHI" IN CHIRUNNING

I'm sure you've seen people who have the uncanny ability to perform at a skill level leagues beyond their nearest peer. They're the ones who can make a difficult activity look like child's play. Anyone who has that high level of connection to the body is doing it by directing chi, whether or not they know it. It might have come easily to them, but it's a highly developed skill nonetheless. A few people of this caliber come to mind for me. One of my favorite people to watch is Barry Sanders, a running back for the Detroit Lions. He could weave his way to the goal line through a crowd of three-hundred-pound people who were totally bent on his demise, making it look like everyone else was in slow motion. He had the focus of a heat-seeking missile and the lightness of a cat. He could change directions quicker than one thought humanly possible, and I loved to watch him stay on his feet and keep his balance through what seemed like unearthly challenges. Even though he probably didn't think about using chi to make his way to the goal line, he was a master at moving his body with the focus and speed of his mind; very much a principle straight out of T'ai Chi.

Barry Sanders, Serena Williams, Yo-Yo Ma, Mikhail Baryshnikov, Marion Jones, Dustin Hoffman, Tiger Woods—the people who might make you say, "Wow, it's unbelievable what they can do with their bodies! How do they do that and make it look so damned easy?" My understanding of how they do it is that they don't *do* anything. They simply get themselves out of the way and allow something else to happen. Not everyone on this list is an athlete, but each is highly skilled in his or her craft to the point of making it an art form. Their high level of skill allows them to cross into realms of physical expression and movement beyond where most of us are capable of going. They can go there because they no longer need to think about what they have to do in the midst of a challenge. When their mind moves, their body follows. If their focus moves, their chi goes with it, and everything that needs to happen takes place as it should, without the interference of doubt, anxiety, tension, fears, or ego, which could dampen the actions of those less skilled in their craft.

Every week when I get to meet Master Xu for another lesson, he gives me example after example of how the power of chi is stronger than muscle. Over and over without using any visible physical effort, he tosses my body around like I'm a feather. His muscles don't tense up as he moves me. He's just moving his body as if I'm not there, and if my body happens to be in the path of his arm, I get flattened. He never breaks a sweat or even breathes hard. All he says is, "I let chi do it." Then he says, "Just set up your body correctly, and let the chi move through it. Let your mind do the work . . . let your body relax. Don't let muscles do it. Let chi do it."

Chi (pronounced *chee*) is also known as life force. It generates movement in the physical world, and it animates life. It is also the energy that is created by movement, so it is both the product and the tool. It is the life-giving energy that unites body, mind, and spirit. An invisible and unmeasurable force that can be seen only by its effect, it is much like air, which can be seen only when it blows through the leaves of a tree or inflates a balloon.

I love to garden, but like any other gardener, I can't make the plants grow. The best I can do is provide the optimal conditions for growth to happen. I can plant the seed in a place that gets good sunlight, and I can add compost to condition the soil, and I can make sure there's plenty of water to nourish the young seedling. Each of these steps helps to ensure that chi will infuse the seed with enough life force to sprout. Somewhere in a desert, a seed can lie dormant for thousands of years in a clay pot at the bottom of an Indian ruin. But it won't sprout unless there is enough chi to get things moving. That's my job as a gardener—to set up the right conditions. The same holds true for ChiRunning. Your job is to learn to set up the optimal conditions for chi to move through your body, and voilà . . . running happens!

THE CHIRUNNING METHOD
AND MIND-SET

Here are the optimal conditions for running and the fundamentals of the ChiRunning method:

- Great posture
- Relaxed limbs
- Loose joints
- Engaged core muscles
- A focused mind
- Good breathing technique

Here are the benefits of using the ChiRunning method:

- Great posture
- Relaxed limbs
- Loose joints
- Engaged core muscles
- A focused mind
- Good breathing technique
- More energy!

You see? The *process* is the goal! There are many more great benefits of ChiRunning, but I just want to make the point that the ChiRunning method is holistic, which means that each of the components contributes positively to the whole by supporting the others to do their job. This aspect of the ChiRunning method also says that you don't have to become an expert in all of the components right away. I've had clients benefit enormously from just one hour of learning how to improve their posture. Any single component will benefit your running, and when all of the components are working together, the effects can be nothing short of transformational.

It's hard to imagine that one could get injured from doing anything on the above list. None of these fundamentals will injure you. And because it's nearly impossible to *overdo* any of them, there is not a downside.

As you learn to incorporate the ChiRunning method into your running, you will dramatically reduce your dependence on strong leg muscles. Gravity will pull you forward, and your speed will be a function of your ability to relax more deeply, not your ability to push harder. I call it "smart effort."

I really don't have any huge desire to spend endless hours building and maintaining muscles, then drinking protein shakes to feed those hungry muscles, then taking ibuprofen to relieve sore muscles—so I've decided to work my *mind* instead.

The ChiRunning mind-set teaches you to listen and focus internally rather than on arbitrary, external goals. The mind-set of ChiRunning is based on establishing a clear and unbroken link of communication between your body and your mind, whereby the process becomes the goal. Your body becomes both your teacher and your pupil. If you pay close attention to it, you can learn what it can and can't do. With that knowledge, you can then teach it new skills and habits. Feel and see where your body is at in the moment, then respond accordingly, in the moment. It is called Body Sensing, and I will tell you more about this skill in Chapter 3. ChiRunning teaches you to be a master of your own body and your own best coach.

There is such cultural pressure in our society to be athletic and have a perfect body. Many people have a negative self-image because they don't see themselves as athletes, even though they might walk or run four days a week. This negative self-image stops people from listening to the messages that their bodies are trying to convey. As I watch beginning runners study their own movements and make necessary corrections, I often see a smile of self-confidence spreading across their face.

Shirlee, 56 (along with many of my clients), has always felt badly about herself because she breathes hard when she runs. She was so embarrassed about her heavy breathing that she wasn't able to focus in class. When she finally confided in me, I was able to give her some tools that helped her to breathe more efficiently. Now her focus is on breathing correctly instead of being embarrassed!

The ChiRunning mind-set is like a dance between your mind and your body—a delightfully cooperative tango. There is a two-way conversation happening all the time between the partners, a constant flow in the moment to create the best conditions for harmonious movement.

THE ROLE OF PHYSICS IN CHIRUNNING

Although I love to study the laws of Nature as reflected in T'ai Chi, I am also a pragmatist. I like to understand how things work on the physical level. In 1999, as I taught a group of scientists at NASA, I discussed the scientific aspects of ChiRunning. They confirmed that the ChiRunning technique is backed by the laws of physics. One scientist even told me, "I wouldn't do this if it didn't work in terms of physics. It makes perfect sense to me, as a scientist." When your body is out of sync with these laws, it becomes less efficient, requires more fuel, experiences greater fatigue, and is more susceptible to injury. Throughout this book I will reference the wisdom of the great T'ai Chi masters as well as the knowledge of the great physicists.

ChiRunning employs physics to correct a number of poor habits of movement that plague most runners. Here are a couple of examples of not making the best use of physics: If you run with your body upright and vertical, like most running coaches will tell you to do, your body is much like a telephone pole—straight up and down, with its centerline plumb with the pull of gravity. If you then want to move your body forward, there are only two ways to make it happen: You can either have a friend push you, or you can push yourself with your legs. Then there's a third way, used in ChiRunning, in which you let your body tilt forward. This will engage the pull of gravity to move you forward, which all but eliminates the need for you to push with your legs. Remember, we're talking about a big paradigm shift here.

Another example of how physics can be used is in your arm swing. Your arm is nothing more than a pendulum that hangs from your shoulder. The law of the pendulum says that the rate at which it swings is directly proportional to its length. If a pendulum is longer, it will swing more slowly, and vice versa, if it is shorter it will swing faster. Running with your hands hanging at your sides means you have to work harder to swing your arms, because your pendulum (arm) is longer. Whereas, if you bend your elbows when you run, you shorten the length of your pendulum, and it will swing faster. The same rule applies to your legs, which are also pendulums. So, bend your elbows and knees, and you'll be able to swing your arms and legs more quickly *and* easily.

Many laws of physics will work to move your body, but some methods of movement are more efficient than others. ChiRunning uses the principles of physics that create the greatest outcome from the least effort, which allows you to run without expending every last drop of energy during your workout. It lets you save some for yourself. Doesn't that sound nice?

DISCOVERY AND UNFOLDMENT

One of the great joys of teaching ChiRunning is seeing people experience running, and themselves, in a way they never imagined. Time after time people have expressed sheer wonder at how great they feel running. From people who were told they could never run again, to complete beginners with little self-confidence, to accomplished runners looking to improve their race times, ChiRunning has had amazing results.

It works because all of the underlying principles are based on moving within the laws of Nature. When you learn to listen to your body, nothing is forced and everything progresses as it should, with little disruption. Ultimately, this approach to running, based on self-discovery and the natural unfoldment of your potential, offers you an opportunity to develop a richer relationship to your body and your Being.

ChiRunning takes you into new territory where running is no longer externally driven, but internally motivated. The emphasis is no longer on increasing speed or distance; those are by-products of sound, efficient running form. You speed demons out there can rest assured that there need be no sacrifice in speed or distance. In fact, it's quite the opposite, if you're so inclined. You can run faster and farther than ever, with less effort and little or no harm to your body. Those of you who aren't speed demons can enjoy being self-respecting athletes at any age or any skill level. The goal is to run freely and joyfully for the rest of your life, and enjoy the full range of benefits that running offers, physically and mentally, and yes, spiritually.

A Comparison: ChiRunning Versus Power Running

CHIRUNNING	POWER RUNNING
Low injury rate	High injury rate
Based on core muscle strength	Based on peripheral (arm and leg) muscle strength
Based on learning to relax muscles instead of using them	Based on strength training
Biomechanics supported by the laws of physics, not the laws of strength	The only biomechanics that are taught are those that support high muscle usage
Requires less fuel	Requires more fuel
Requires little or no recovery time between workouts	Requires more recovery time
Requires use of ligaments and tendons instead of muscles	Main focus is on using muscles and strength to power one's movement
Creates less impact on the body	High impact
Muscle cells are not broken down during training	Muscle cells are broken down during training in order to be rebuilt as larger muscles (the body's ability to produce muscle cells diminishes with age)
Looser joints have less injury potential	Overdeveloped muscles create tight joints, which are then vulnerable to impact
Less is more	Bigger is better
Process-oriented	Goal-oriented
No pain, no pain	No pain, no gain

CHAPTER TWO

The Principles of ChiRunning: Moving with Nature

Principles are deep fundamental truths that have universal application. Principles are guidelines for human conduct that are proven to have enduring, permanent value. —STEVEN COVEY

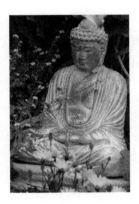

ChiRunning is based on a set of principles that will help you run, and train, in a more effortless and efficient way. These principles are a huge part of my regular T'ai Chi lessons with Master Xu and have had a profound impact on me, not only in how I move my body but in how I view the world.

Thousands of years ago, Chinese masters studied how Nature works and defined these principles in writings such as the Tao Te Ching (the most widely translated book besides the Bible), the I Ching (the preeminent book of Chinese philosophy), and in the practice of T'ai Chi (the mother of martial arts, which dates back over 2,500 years). But it's not just the Chinese who have studied these principles. Guys like Einstein and Newton defined many of them as the laws of physics.

It is no wonder people of deep wisdom and intellect chose to study Nature. It has a set of basic principles that seem to work pretty well. Anyone can see how perfectly Nature operates when left to itself. Everything in Nature has a deep sense of order and rightness. It is harmonious. You don't find animals out of place, and plants don't grow where the conditions are not right. Even on the molecular level, everything has an order and a place, and somehow it's all held in balance. It all works!

These laws can also be thought of as universal laws. For a law to be universal, it has to hold true on all four basic levels of existence: physical, emotional, mental, and spiritual. For instance, one law says, "A body at rest tends to remain at rest unless acted upon by an external force."

Here are some examples of how this law works on different levels:

- On the physical level: A couch potato won't move unless either the power goes off and the TV goes blank or he runs out of chips.
- On the mental level: It's a philosophical change, such as when Christopher Columbus came along and discovered the New World.
- On an emotional level: I can go through an entire day absorbed in my own drama, until my daughter throws her arms around my neck and says, "I love you, Daddy," which zaps me out of my brain and into my heart.
- On a spiritual level: It might take a near-death experience for someone to realize how precious life really is.

The beauty of universal laws is that when you learn a law on one level, it can show you how life works on other levels.

What Happens When You Resist or Don't Follow the Law?

Well, I can pretty safely say the consequence of breaking a universal law is more than just paying a fine and promising not to do it again. It will increase your workload in the short term and will inevitably lead to some level of failure in the long term. In your running, you may have more speed, but you'll have a beat-up body. You may have a good race but feel like hell the next day. Working against the laws of physics requires you to rely more on your own strength than on the forces of Nature.

Running can be in harmony with the laws of nature, but power running is not. Over 15 million people in the U.S. alone getting injured every year should be cause for alarm. No wonder *Sports Injury Bulletin* classifies running as a high-injury sport. The questions that this brings up are: (1) Should people be running? And (2) Is there a better way?

For question 1, the answer is yes: Our physiology is well suited for running. We were designed to run. As for question 2, from my own experience with ChiRunning and having taught it to thousands of people, I can say, unequivocally, yes, there is a better way.

Have you ever tried to swim upstream? You can do it if you're strong enough. And if you're not strong enough, you can work hard and build big muscles so that you can eventually do it. But no matter how you look at it, you're swimming against the current, and that's going to take a lot of work. I mean, salmon do it, but they die when they get there. So, as long as you're in the water, you have to follow the law of the water. On the other hand, if you want to get upstream with less effort, simply get out of the water and into a different set of laws, where getting upstream might involve nothing more than a gentle walk up a fern-lined path. As Cecil B. DeMille said regarding his epic film, *The Ten Commandments,* "It is impossible for us to break the law ourselves. We can only break ourselves against the law."

GOING WITH THE FLOW

When you are working within natural laws, there is less effort involved and less of the physical breakdown experienced with power running. When you run economically, you don't require as much fuel to keep going, you don't get tired as easily, and it doesn't take as long to recover from your runs. When you are not overworking your muscles and joints, there will be less chance for injury. When you cooperate with universal law, you become powerful on all levels, including attitude. You will be able to go out for a run and come back feeling better than when you took off.

The Key Principles

Here are the key principles on which ChiRunning is based. In this chapter I'll go over their definitions, and in Chapter 4, I'll break down the principles into very specific focuses and exercises that will help you move your body in a more fluid, efficient, and graceful way, one step at a time. The five key principles are:

- **(I) Cotton and Steel:** Gather to Your Center
- **(II) Gradual Progress:** The Step-by-Step Approach
- **(III) The Pyramid:** The Small Is Supported by the Large
- **(IV) Balance in Motion:** Equal Balance and Complementary Balance
- **(V) Nonidentification:** Getting Yourself Out of the Way

As you become more adept at practicing and integrating these principles into your running, you will begin to feel an ease in how your body moves. Instead of your body being a tool for running, your running becomes a tool for your body.

Cotton and Steel: Gather to Your Center

This is one of the main principles taught in T'ai Chi. It is considered the foundation of all movement in the body. The phrase "cotton and steel" describes the feeling that a T'ai Chi practitioner should have while doing the form. When you concentrate chi energy to your center, your arms and legs are as soft as cotton, holding no tension.

In ChiRunning, as in T'ai Chi, all movement in your body originates in your center. It is your power source, acting as the axis around which everything else moves. According to T'ai Chi, your center, or *dan tien,* is located just below your navel and in front of your spine. It is conveniently hooked up to your arms and legs by a series of bones, ligaments, and tendons, so whenever you move your center, your arms and legs move, too. But in order for your center to do its work efficiently, the rest of your body has to relax and offer no resistance to the movement.

The emphasis in ChiRunning is on learning how to run from your center, and the better you get at that, the less you need your legs to run. I know that sounds counterintuitive, but it's true. When Master Xu is teaching me to move, he has me gather my energy and mental focus into my *dan tien* while softening the rest of my body so that it will be moved by my center and not by my muscles. When I move in this way, I can feel the fluidity in my gait led by the movement in my center.

When you run from a place outside your center, it is less powerful because you are doing so from an unbalanced state. Your legs have to work many times harder than if the rest of your body were helping out. When you don't run from your center, your running form is not "organized," because your arms and legs and trunk are moving as three independent entities instead of one harmonious, fluid unit. I have observed many runners who are moving their arms and legs and going through the motions of running, but what is missing is the sense of integrity that comes from having a strong center.

Our Milky Way has a center around which all the stars in the galaxy rotate. Our solar system has a center, the sun, around which all the planets rotate. Our earth also has a center, and it spins on an axis that runs right through it. Our country has a center that is said to be somewhere in Missouri, although I've never been there. In the ChiRunning technique, it all begins by learning to locate and sense your center when you run.

Try this sampling: Stand up straight, with your best posture and one foot slightly behind the other, hip width apart. Relax your shoulders and let your arms hang limp at your sides. Now pretend that your spine is a vertical axle. Let it rotate first in one direction and then in the other. As you rotate your spine back and forth, your arms will move because your spine is moving; let them flail against your body in a gentle way. Focus on keeping your spine straight while rotating back and forth. Stay with the image of your spine being an axle. Try to see how relaxed you can make your shoulders, arms, and wrists. This is an example of your core doing the work while your arms are just along for the ride.

Here is a visualization to practice anytime during the day and as often as possible. Imagine a line between the top of your head and your tailbone. This is your centerline. Keep it in your mind's eye when you are walking or running. Start by focusing on it while you're standing still. Become friends with it and remember it. Make it as familiar as your breath. Don't try to do anything with it. Just acknowledge it. See it. Learn that it is a location within your body.

Find your center in your body.
Sense your center in your feelings.
See your center in your mind.
Be centered in your spirit.

Gradual Progress: The Step-by-Step Approach

The Gradual Progress principle says that everything has to grow incrementally through its own developmental stages, from less to more or from smaller to larger. When a growth process happens gradually, each step forms a stable foundation for the next step. This principle holds true for any growth process, whether it's an object, an idea, a feeling, or a life form. An example on the physical plane would be a tree growing from a seed. It starts off small and gets larger as the cells divide and multiply. Another example would be a business start-up: The owner begins a business from an idea that develops into a plan that leads to opening its doors to the public. The business would start off small, and if the owner did things right, it would grow into a thriving business.

If you try to break this law and skip steps, you'll encounter either a negative effect on the process or a diminished outcome. Consider the terminal torrid love affair, in which two people meet and instantly have the hots for each other. They spend the next four nights joined at the hip and then skip off to Las Vegas to get married. Then they file for a divorce after about three weeks because they forgot to build a friendship.

As you may have already guessed, a big factor in the success of this principle is time. Lots of people come to me and say they'd like to run a marathon. The first question I ask them is "How long is your current long run?" If they answer with a distance under 10K, my next question is "Which year would you like to run it?" Running a marathon is not that hard to do if you take plenty of time to slowly build up your mileage. The first race I trained for and ran was a 50-mile race. That may seem really far for a first race, and it was. But I trained for three and a half years to do it. I started off with a 10-mile long run and increased my mileage only when it felt right. Building up slowly allowed my body to adjust to the increasing mileage. It allowed me to take the time to correct imperfections in my form that were causing me pain. But most of all, it allowed me to gradually build the confidence that running 50 miles didn't have to be a big deal or harmful to my body.

I witness runners breaking this rule most often on race day. Everyone lines up at the starting line, and when the gun fires, they take off as if the finish line were at the end of the block. If I stick around for the finish of the race, I usually see the familiar faces of those rabbits who shot away from the starting line, only now they look a little like a bad guy in a western movie, staggering forward after being shot in the back.

Sorry, folks, but I can't pass up one more example. Remember all those dot-coms that used to be in business in the 1990s? Let's just say they went out a little too fast at the starting gate and paid the price of breaking this law.

This scenario happens a lot in power running. The basic script is: (1) Train hard for the race. (2) Once you start the race, run as fast as you can and hang on to whatever speed you can until your fuel runs out. (3) Try to get across the finish line without losing that bagel you slam-dunked on your way out of the house.

The principle of Gradual Progress is always applied in ChiRunning, whether it's a single run or a running program. When starting a run, it's important to start slowly, and pick up the speed as your body adapts to the movement of running. Just as you wouldn't drive off from a stoplight in fourth gear, you wouldn't start a run or a running program too fast. Instead, you accelerate through the gears until you reach your cruising speed. Your body is no exception. Don't start a running program with too much speed or mileage or you could get injured. Most training injuries happen when someone's ego starts getting ahead of the rate at which his body can produce new muscle cells. For something to end up solid, it has to grow step by step and move through all of the sequential stages of growth. If you start skipping steps, you're breaking this law, and the consequences can range from fatigue to aches to injuries. Sixty percent of all running injuries occur because of overtraining, which means either too much mileage or too fast an upgrade in speed or mileage. On the emotional level, if you start off a program too fast and burn out because of the intensity, you could end up not even wanting to go out and run. I'll use this principle extensively in Chapter 6.

If I break this law when I'm running, I pay in one form or another. I end up with a slower time, sore legs, longer recovery, or even injury. When I start off too fast with an activity in my life, I increase my odds of failure or disappointment. Go step by step, gradually increase, and let each new stage be built on what you've learned from the preceding stages. Gradual Progress—it's a law we can live with.

THE PYRAMID: THE SMALL IS SUPPORTED BY THE LARGE

Try this exercise: Stand up and run in place for 10 seconds. Next pick up your feet for 10 seconds (as if you're walking in place). Now go back to running in place for another 10 seconds, then walk in place for 10 seconds. Go ahead . . . do it, and then come back to the book.

I want you to tell me. Which would be easier to do for two hours:

(A) picking up your feet
   or
(B) running in place?

If you picked A, go to the head of the class. If you picked B, go back and repeat the exercise for two hours.

I have all my beginning running classes do this exercise, and when they've finished picking up their feet in place, I ask them this question. Out of about 3,000 runners I've asked, I've had a handful say they'd choose to run in place for the two hours. The other 2,997 easily agreed that they would rather pick up their feet, because it felt like less work.

Here's what happens in this exercise. When you run in place, the last part of your body to leave the ground is the ball of your foot. If you stand up right now on the balls of your feet, you'll notice that your calves tighten. When you run in place, your calves (a relatively small muscle group, compared to the quads) are being used to propel the weight of your body into the air. That's *hard* work. If you really did run in place this way for two hours, I could almost guarantee that your perceived effort level would be off the charts, and you'd end up with a major case of shin splints.

On the other hand, if you're picking up your feet, you're using your psoas muscles and hip flexors. Those are two of the strongest core muscles in your body, working to lift the weight of your feet, which means that there's a *large* muscle group doing a *tiny* job. That's why your PEL drops into the minimal range. If you could run by just picking up your feet, why would you want to push your weight around all day, wearing yourself out? If you sense in your body that picking up your feet is the easier way to go, that's because it is.

Here are some examples of this principle:

- Build a solid base in your running program, and it will make each individual run go easier.
- The president has a lot more power to enact change if the House and Senate back him up.

- Supportive parents make a huge difference in helping a child to become a self-confident adult.
- Work from your center and let your core do the bulk of the work, so your arms and legs can relax.
- Everything and everyone needs support. No man—or woman, for that matter—is an island.

The Pyramid principle allows you to be very efficient in your movement and economical in your energy consumption. This can translate into being able to run faster or farther, because you are not using up your available fuel at a disproportionate rate. It's all about energy conservation. If your small muscles are doing big work, they use up your energy at a higher rate than if the right muscle is doing the right job. Another place where this principle needs to operate is in your running program. Each progressive stage should have a solid foundation in the training that comes before.

One day Master Xu was trying to get me to sense this principle at work. He held his arm out in front of his body and told me to push on it as hard as I could while he tried to hold me off: "First, I'm going to hold you off with my muscles." Which he did, and it was pretty much a standoff. I could feel his body tensing and his arm quivering to hold back my body weight as I pushed him as hard as I could.

"Now I'm going to push against you again," he said calmly. This time I might as well have been a paper cup that he was knocking off a picnic table. I flew about ten feet backward, struggling to land somewhat upright. What happened? I had been totally taken by surprise. He hadn't tensed his muscles or winced or given me any indication that I was about to be launched. He just moved his arm as if I wasn't there!

When I asked him how he did it, he replied, "I just relaxed my body and let the chi of the neighborhood behind me push you. Big thing do big job." No kidding.

Your core muscles work your hips and shoulders. Your hips and shoulders move your arms and legs. Your arms and legs move your wrists and ankles, and they in turn move your fingers and toes. None of these should be out of order, or it will cost you energy.

Balance in Motion:
Equal Balance and Complementary Balance

You've probably seen the symbol for yin/yang. It's a circle that is half black and half white, with an S-shaped line separating the two halves. Among other things, it is the symbol of balance. But unlike a circle with a line straight down the middle, dividing the figure into two equal halves, the shape represents complementary energy balance. Notice that as one portion of the circle gets larger, the section of the circle on the other side of the line gets smaller. Whenever one side is expanded, the other side is contracted. When one side is hard, one side is soft. When one side is light, the other side is heavy. Balance doesn't always mean equal balance. It means that in order for something to increase, something else has to decrease, and vice versa.

HOW IT WORKS IN RUNNING

In your running, you need to balance your movement and effort. In ChiRunning, as in T'ai Chi, the balance happens in six directions: left to right, up to down, and front to back. As one part of your body moves forward, its complement moves to the rear. As your body leans forward, your stride opens up out the back. Whenever one side of your body is extending, the other side is gathering.

If you run with just your legs, without bringing in all the help from the rest of the body, then you're running in an unbalanced state, and your legs will be overworked. If you have a heavy rock to move, it's much easier to get five people to do it so the workload gets spread out. ChiRunning is a way to run with all of your body engaged in a unified way, each part doing its proportional share. When all parts are working in harmony, your body moves in a balanced way. When a cheetah runs, there is no part of its body that isn't contributing to the effort, and its running is balanced.

Here are a few examples of how balance can manifest itself:

- Balance of fluids: The more you sweat, the more you need to drink.
- Balance of workouts: Alternate easy and hard workouts.
- Balance of fuel: The harder you work, the more fuel you require.
- Balance of effort: The faster you run, the more you need to relax your legs.
- Balance of work and play: The harder you work, the more important it is that you play.

NONIDENTIFICATION: GETTING YOURSELF OUT OF THE WAY

This principle addresses the theme of Moving with Nature. When you put your personal preferences aside and align yourself with natural laws, then things happen as they should. When your ego gets in there and wants to control the outcome or the process, it throws you out of sync with how events naturally unfold. Another common phrase is: "Go with the flow." When I'm out trail running, for instance, I try to let the terrain tell my body what to do instead of gutting it out on the steep ups and downs. I can run much better and more efficiently if I go with the flow of the trail instead of fighting it. When I'm running up a steep hill, I don't get bummed out that there's a lot of work ahead. I relax my legs, which shortens my stride, making the hill easier to negotiate. It's like downshifting in your car. Nature is telling me that it takes smaller steps to do bigger work. I don't resist the hill; I make friends with it and let it show me what to do. Likewise, when I'm running downhill, I pretend I'm a stream flowing along taking the most efficient path. If I fight the steepness of the trail, my leg muscles will tense, and I'll feel the crushing impact of my body weight every time my foot meets the earth. Whereas, if I can relax my body and legs, I feel more like a lowrider cruising East L.A. on a Saturday night than a Jeep pounding my way over each rock and root in my path.

Getting yourself out of the way also means making friends with injuries and letting them tell you what you're doing wrong. When people tell me that they've had a bad run, it's music to my ears. If I ask the right questions about why they considered the run bad, I can pinpoint the weak spot in their technique and guide them to the necessary correction. If you look at your challenging or difficult runs in this way, you won't be as compelled to call them "bad runs." Instead, you could tell your friends that you had a good "running lesson" today.

CONCLUSION

Until we move with Nature and don't try to force our bodies against natural laws, our forward progress will forever be met with resistance in the form of injury, fatigue, disappointment, or plain old difficulty. When you allow yourself to be guided by these principles, running becomes a way to create health for your whole being, and any doubts about whether or not running is good for you will evaporate. With the power of Nature backing you up, the potential for success and enjoyment is vast.

CHAPTER THREE

The Four Chi-Skills

How do you best move toward mastery? To put it simply, you practice diligently, but you practice primarily for the sake of the practice itself.—GEORGE LEONARD, *MASTERY*

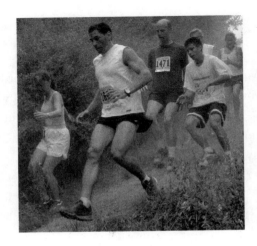

I spent fifteen years as a woodworker, learning the value of always working to improve one's skill level. Whenever I made a costly miscalculation, I was forced to call on ingenuity and skill to pull me out of the fire. I can honestly say that I learned more skills from the countless mistakes I made than from all the woodworking books on my shelf. I was also blessed to have some highly talented mentors teaching me the resourcefulness to turn a tree into a finely crafted piece of furniture.

Craftsmen and artisans depend on their skills to see them through any challenge that might arise. It is no different with running, or with life, for that matter. My two seemingly disparate fields of interest share the same four underlying skills, which I call Chi-Skills: Focusing, Body Sensing, Breathing, and Relaxing.

The Chi-Skills are my essential tools for running that I'd like to share with you. There is no question that when I run a 50K race, I am using all of these skills to maximize performance while minimizing physical effort. The use of Chi-Skills allows your running to become multidimensional. Your workouts will have more depth and breadth because there's something more going on than running. You will begin to approach running in ways that go beyond the realms of farther or faster.

These skills will help you reach any goal in life with greater ease. Although we all use them every day, we often do so unconsciously. By consciously practicing Chi-Skills in your running, you will increase your capacity to focus your mind, sense your body, relax (don't most of us have trouble with this important skill?), and maximize the benefits of the most basic of acts—breathing.

As always in ChiRunning, the process is the goal. Chi-Skills are both valuable skills and worthwhile goals at the same time. So, every time you practice focusing your mind, you are accomplishing your goal of being more focused. It is a very satisfying effort.

In Chapter 7 we will go into details of how to incorporate the Chi-Skills and the technique focuses into your running program. But for now, practicing any of these skills for five minutes on a run, or while doing practically anything (from washing dishes to changing a diaper) will increase your capability with that skill and also improve the caliber of your run or activity. These skills improve the quality of your running *and* the quality of your life.

FOCUSING YOUR MIND

ChiRunning is the thinking person's way to run. There will probably never be a "ChiRunning for Dummies." Although it's important for people to get a physical experience first, it is the mind that really does the bulk of the work in ChiRunning. Your mind turns off the chatter and focuses so it can listen to your body. Your mind instructs your muscles to start working or relaxing. Your mind orchestrates the perfect run, starting out slowly, finding the perfect tempo, and taking in the beauty and chi of your surroundings so that you finish relaxed, empowered, and full of energy for the day ahead.

There are many worthwhile reasons to learn something new, whether it's ChiRunning, a foreign language, a musical instrument, or a new recipe. Learning is what we are meant to do. It is our birthright as humans. If we stop learning, we stop growing, and our minds become stagnant. If you don't use it, you'll lose it.

Two of the key ingredients (and great benefits) of learning and practicing ChiRunning are a focused mind and a responsive body. When your mind is focused and your body is responsive, you have y'chi (pronounced *ee-chee*), a full mind/body focus. It's the unbreakable focus of a cat when it stalks a bird, or a tennis player awaiting a serve, or a meter maid while she's writing you a parking ticket.

Think of your own experiences of y'chi. We've all had them in our lives. Perhaps it was when you first met the love of your life; your whole focus was probably consumed by that person. Perhaps it was when you gave a major presentation to an important client, or when you flipped your first egg without breaking it. It could have been when you discovered your life's work, or perhaps it was as simple as trying to sink a thirty-foot putt on the eighteenth hole of the final round of the PGA with a thousand spectators breathlessly awaiting the tap.

"But who wants to focus that much?" you might ask. "I just run to relax and rest my mind." Like a meditation practice, the training of the mind and body in ChiRunning is more relaxing than letting the mind wander. Studies have shown that watching TV is not as relaxing as sitting quietly. A focused mind is more relaxed than a mind that wanders aimlessly through the details and minutiae of the day. When you are focused on teaching yourself something new, the benefits to your body and mind will far outweigh the effort it takes to focus. Eventually, as the ChiRunning form becomes second nature, your mind and body become as one. It is no longer *work* to focus your mind. It is not even a thought process, because the situation and the response are simultaneous. Like the cat stalking the bird, you're pulled forward by your y'chi. Practicing the ChiRunning focuses is preparation for developing and utilizing your y'chi in any situation.

Bob, age 48, had been a recreational runner for 15 years when he came to his first ChiRunning class. He told me that he had gone out 5 days a week for the past 3 years and run a 3-mile loop around his neighborhood like clockwork. He had done it so regularly that he knew within seconds how long it would take him to arrive back at his own front door. After attending the ChiRunning clinic, he went out the next day, armed with all of the focuses that he could remember, and proceeded to run his loop as usual. He was used to coming home feeling a distinct sense of having done his obligatory exercise for the day. This day, when he arrived back at his house, he looked at his watch, expecting to see the usual numbers. To his surprise, his time was 3 minutes faster than his previous best. He told me he thought his watch had stopped during the run, so he tapped on it to make sure it was working. Not only that, he wasn't at all tired. In fact, he felt so good that he immediately went out and ran another 2 miles! He had done so well at keeping his mind attentive to the focuses that his body could simply relax and go along for the ride!

Keeping the ChiRunning focuses can be a meditative practice that trains your mind to curtail its arbitrary wanderings. As in meditation, the greater aspect of ChiRunning is that you learn how to be present with your mind and body, which is where true inner freedom lies.

If all you want to do is learn to run without injuring yourself, or perhaps get a little faster or run longer, ChiRunning can get you there. If you're also interested in the benefits of meditation and the power of a focused mind, ChiRunning can offer you that as well. For it is a focused mind moving with the relaxed, responsive body that does, in the end, give you the ease of movement you're looking for.

If you'd like a sample of what it feels like to focus your mind, try this: Sit up straight in your chair and hold your best posture while you read the rest of this chapter. Don't let yourself slouch even once. That's it! Your focus is to maintain good posture. I'll ask you at the end of this chapter how you did.

BODY SENSING: HIGH-SPEED ACCESS

Body Sensing is the act of feeling what's going on inside of your body. When you swing your leg, what does it feel like? Does it feel right?

Could it feel better, easier, smoother, more relaxed? When you take an action, Body Sensing is the voice of your body. When your mind gives a directive to your body, it will respond with a movement, and Body Sensing will tell you the effectiveness of that response. Body Sensing will tell you when you're working too hard or not enough. It can tell you when to add some muscle to what you are doing and when to take it away.

Body Sensing is the link between your body and your mind, and chi makes that connection possible. It is the substance that travels through your "phone lines," and the more you practice using this medium, the clearer the connection gets.

When I was a kid, my brother and I used to play telephone with two tin cans and a piece of wire. It was primitive, but it got the basic job of communication done. Now I have a computer with a cable modem, and I can send e-mail, recordings, snapshots, and movies. There are many methods available today, but the bottom line is good clear communication.

The tin cans have many parallels to Body Sensing. When I first started to run, many years ago, it was on the tin-can level: My mind would tell my body to go out and run. Then I would run until my body said it was tired, which would trigger my mind to call it quits for the day. That was the extent of the communication between my body and my mind.

Now that I'm more skilled at Body Sensing, I can give my body very detailed and specific directives and listen for the subtle nuances. Depending on the response, I will either make a needed adjustment or not. Each time I make an adjustment, I listen very carefully with my mind to what my body is telling me. I never judge my body's responses as good or bad. They're just responses, and I'm collecting data. At this point the dialogue between my mind and my body has become deep and clearly understandable, and it goes on all the time, whether I'm running or not. I not only enjoy the interaction, I depend on it. If I listen carefully enough, my body will tell me everything I need to know to create optimal results.

Here is another tin-can analogy. When I talked to my brother through that primitive wire connection, there was usually so much static on the line that I could barely make out what he was saying. If the wire touched any obstacles between him and me, additional noise would come through the line and garble the main message. Likewise, there are factors that will add "static" to your line, making it difficult to receive a clear message from your body. The static that I'm talking about is generated by your mental activity—your ideas and attitudes about what your body is doing or could be doing. Body Sensing is not a *thinking* process, it's a *sensing* process. Any negative or judgmental thinking makes static on the line, and you don't need that when you're trying to get clear reception. Watch for phrases like "I should" or "I can't" or "I'm not" or "I have to."

Body Sensing is the skill I have used in the *process* of learning and developing ChiRunning, and it has also become an *end* unto itself that is now second nature.

The ChiRunning technique is more than just a running form. It is an activity that works to build a strong link between your mind and body. When learning the ChiRunning technique, you will be asked to move your body in a particular way and then to Body Sense so you can tell if you're running with the correct form. You'll know when you're doing it right, because your running will no longer feel like work. It will take on a new sense of effortlessness.

In Chapter 4 you will learn the ChiRunning form focuses, which are the building blocks of sound, efficient technique. As you practice each of these focuses, you will be setting your body up to experience a new way to run. You will eventually sense an ease in your movement, much like finding the sweet spot in a tennis racket. It is the very distinct feeling of your mind and body working as one.

HOW TO DO BODY SENSING

This is one of my favorite exercises for learning Body Sensing. You will learn will how to tell the difference between perception and reality when it comes to your body—a skill we could all use.

Exercise

Stand in front of a full-length mirror. Now, keeping your eyes closed, position yourself with your feet parallel, your knees slightly bent, shoulders squared, arms and hands relaxed at your sides. Begin by sensing your feet on the ground and the position your feet are in.

Feel your legs.

Feel your hips.

Feel your torso . . .

. . . your arms, hands, shoulders, and the position of your head.

Imagine how you look by how your body feels to you. Spend time really feeling the position of your body. After one minute of doing this, open your eyes.

Note all the differences between how you *thought* your body looked and how your body actually looks in the mirror.

- Are your feet truly parallel?
- Are your shoulders aligned with each other?
- Are your fingers straight or curved?
- Is your head on straight?

Now stand sideways to the mirror, and close your eyes again. Make your feet parallel and stand with your best posture. Again, take 3 minutes to really feel the position of your body. When you open your eyes, you'll have to turn your head and look at yourself from the side. Once again, note the differences between what you felt and what you see in the mirror.

- Is your spine vertical or slumped?
- Is your chin up or down?

Practice this regularly, and you'll become adept at truly sensing the positions of your arms, legs, and body. You'll also become more skilled at directing your body to move as you want it to move.

This exercise is similar to what goes on when I videotape students. They'll think they're running in a certain way, but when they see what they're actually doing, it has a huge impact on their view of themselves. Seeing the "truth" through the eyes of a video camera allows them to make adjustments with a much greater degree of accuracy.

Do this exercise first thing every morning before your day really gets rolling, or whenever you're at the gym, where there's a mirrored wall. The entire exercise should take about 10 minutes. The longer it takes, the better it will work for you. Don't hurry through; take the time to enjoy sensing your body and getting to know it. Faster is not better. Doing this exercise consistently will build in you an ability to sense what is going on anywhere in your body.

Here's a more general "how to" of Body Sensing in three steps. Try to get a sense of what each one means for you. We all speak with our own dialect, so don't feel you have to be rigid with these steps. They're guidelines for how to develop the skill of Body Sensing. You can repeat these steps as many times as needed to effect change.

(1) Listen Carefully

Pay very close attention to what your body is doing. Practice listening to any little nuances that you can detect. How is your body moving, and what does it feel like? What sensations are you noticing in various parts?

(2) Assess the Information

Do your best to discern if any adjustment you're trying to apply is working or not. If it is, then try to physically memorize how it feels and how you got there. If it isn't, then try to sense what doesn't feel quite right.

Here are some questions to ask yourself in evaluating your efforts:

Is your body moving in the way that you intended it to?

Is your movement easier or more difficult?

Is there more or less discomfort?

(3) Adjust Incrementally

Making subtle adjustments is always the best policy. Any abrupt change in how you move your body is an invitation for injury.

You will be learning how to use your mind to set up the ChiRunning form focuses that are the specific parts of the technique. As you work with each of these focuses, you will have to Body Sense whether or not you are doing them correctly. Let's say that your focus is to relax your ankles while you run. First, your mind will tell your ankles to relax. Then you will listen to what your body is doing with the instructions. If you do it right, your ankles will feel soft and loose, in which case you will memorize what it feels like to have relaxed ankles, then you'll duplicate that the next time you go running. If you don't fully relax your ankles, you might experience a pulling sensation in your Achilles tendon, or tightness in your calf muscles. That's your body telling you that relaxation isn't happening. So you make an assessment and ask your body to make the adjustment. It's best to repeat this cycle until you feel satisfied that you're moving correctly, or at least in the right direction.

When you're first learning Body Sensing, it is best to train yourself using outside sources. Ask a friend or running partner to watch you. Tell her what you are trying to do, and ask her if you look like you're doing it. An even better way to see yourself is to have someone videotape you while you run. Then you can play back the tape and either stop the action or slow it down to see the details of how you're moving. This will allow you to make a direct comparison between what you were attempting to do and what you are actually doing. You may think you are leaning when you're not. You may think your arms are swinging like crazy when they're just hanging at your sides. People have their biggest breakthroughs when they see themselves on a videotape replay. This is because they can remember how they *felt* when they were running, then match that up with how they *looked* in the video.

When you get skilled at Body Sensing, you become your own best teacher and coach. Once you get used to always using the three steps of Body Sensing, you'll never be left in the dark, wondering what to do next or whether you're doing something right, because your body will be there to tell you where you are, and your mind will be there to direct you where to go next.

BREATHING: TAPPING INTO YOUR CHI

Breathing is a skill, just like Body Sensing and focusing. It is at the core of many Eastern disciplines, such as yoga, tantra, chi gung, and meditation. There are books written entirely on the breath and the importance of proper breathing technique. Breathing is one way for chi to enter the body. In yoga, breathing practices are called *pranayama, prana* being the equivalent of chi. In running, as in all other types of aerobic exercise, the breath holds the key role of providing oxygen to help fuel active muscles. If you don't get enough oxygen to your muscles, they will be starved of the key component needed for burning fuel. The more efficiently your body can extract oxygen from the air and transfer it to your muscles, the easier your running will feel at any speed. Later in this section I will give you tips on how to improve that efficiency.

Many people experience shortness of breath while running. It's not a bad thing. It's *supposed* to happen, especially if you're running faster or farther than your body is conditioned to go. I've had many people admit that they intentionally taught themselves to breathe slowly so no one would know how out of shape they were; meanwhile, they were killing zillions of brain cells to look good. There are also people who experience a large amount of fear when they start to breathe hard. Heavy breathing brings up everyone's worst nightmares and triggers the negative voices of insecurities, such as:

- I'm going to die.
- I can't keep up.
- I can't do this.
- I'm no good.
- This is hard.
- I'm embarrassed.
- I can't believe I'm so out of shape!

Heavy breathing triggers a sense of running out of air, of suffocating, of passing out due to a lack of oxygen or heart attack.

There are many reasons why you might come up short of breath. I'll discuss a few of them here and do what I can to dispel your fears.

LOW AEROBIC CAPACITY

When you're just starting up a running program, you can expect to be out of breath at first. That's because your muscles are not equipped to take in the additional oxygen supply needed to sustain the increased workload. The best way to increase your aerobic capacity is with LSD. No, it doesn't stand for lysergic acid diethylamide—it stands for *l*ong *s*low *d*istance running. Doing LSD is what helps increase your aerobic capacity. (I'll cover aerobic training in Chapter 6.) Having a long run in your program ensures that your muscles will be able to keep up with the demand for oxygen. The trick to building aerobic capacity is to do your long run at a conversational pace, meaning that you're moving along at a rate that you never come close to feeling out of breath. You should be able to easily carry on a conversation . . . hopefully with whomever is running with you.

SHALLOW BREATHING

If you're breathing from the upper part of your lungs, you're not getting as much air as you could. A doctor in one of my classes assured me that there are no alveoli (those little sacs in your lungs that extract the oxygen from the air) in your upper lungs. Therefore, if you're breathing into only your upper lungs, you're not getting as much air into your blood supply, even though you might be breathing like a freight train. The cure for this is to breathe deeply, into your lower lungs. If you're short of breath, it's not because you aren't breathing *in* enough—it's because you're not breathing *out* enough. It is important to fully empty your lungs from the bottom, so the used air can be expelled completely, thereby allowing a fresh supply of oxygen back in.

Here's how to belly-breathe: Stand or sit and place your hands over your belly button. Now purse your lips as if you're trying to blow a candle out, and exhale, emptying your lungs by pulling in your belly button toward your spine. When you've blown out as much air as you can, relax your belly, and the inhale will occur naturally. If you want to get additional air into your lungs, you can expand your lower rib cage as you inhale. Practice breathing this way when you're not running, so you can learn the technique without being under physical duress. Once you get comfortable with belly breathing, you can introduce it into your running. Try matching up your breathing with your cadence. I usually breathe out for three steps and breathe in for two, but do what works best for you. It helps if you take more time breathing out than breathing in.

CARRYING TENSION IN YOUR MUSCLES

If your muscles are tight or tense, it is much more difficult for oxygen to squeeze its way into your muscle cells, because the oxygenated blood from your lungs cannot enter dense (tense) muscles. It's like the difference between pouring syrup on pancakes or dumping it on bagels. The bagels are so dense that they don't absorb anything, while the pancakes are more like sponges.

The cure for this is easy. Just relax! Isn't that why you're running to begin with? Don't take yourself so seriously. Drop your shoulders. Smile. Relax your glutes; don't be a tight-ass. Float like a butterfly . . . lighten up!

YOU JUST ATE A HUGE DINNER, YOUR 3-YEAR-OLD WANTS TO PLAY TAG, AND YOU FEEL LIKE A BEACHED WHALE

There is no cure for this. Just have fun and do your best to hold on to that dinner.

I've seen runners who have increased their speed and distance simply by learning to breathe right. The better you get at identifying your reason for shortness of breath, the sooner you'll be able to do something about it. Running regularly with a long slow run once a week will ensure that you're building the necessary aerobic capacity. The biggest help to your breathing will be when you learn to really relax while you're running. Then everything happens more easily. Because you're working more efficiently, your oxygen requirements are lower, and your breathing will take on more of a natural rhythm.

Proper breathing is touted as an aid to everything from better vision and brainpower to better sex. There is no end to the value of working with your breath, and with the few suggestions described here, you should be breathing well and easy no matter what your undertaking. Now set this book down in your lap, sit up straight, take a deep breath, and let out a big "AHHHHHHHHHHHHH." See? It's not that hard to breathe well. You just have to remind yourself to do it.

RELAXATION: THE PATH OF LEAST RESISTANCE

I don't know anybody who couldn't stand to have a little more relaxation in his life, me included. But as paradoxical as it sounds, we all have to *work* to make it happen. Interestingly enough, the three best tools to help you learn to relax are: Focusing, Body Sensing, and Breathing, which is why relaxation completes the list of Chi-Skills.

Almost everyone I know lives in some state of density, where there is always a little more going on than we'd like. We all need and crave some *spaciousness* in our lives, whether it's figurative or literal. I use the image of spaciousness while I'm running. I imagine having openness in my joints and lots of ease in my motion. Nothing feels forced. My movement is free and loose. Now, *that's* the kind of relaxation that I'm talking about.

Master Xu was helping me through yet another T'ai Chi lesson and moving his body without apparently using his muscles. His arms were moving, but his muscles were limp and flaccid. He said to me, "Here, rest your hand on my arm, and keep it there while I go through this movement." I did as he asked.

"Now I'm moving my arm using my muscles," he said, smiling. Indeed he was. I could feel the strength in his forearm. Firm and rigid, it felt like an overdone drumstick at Thanksgiving dinner.

"Now I'm moving with my chi," he said, smiling even more broadly.

Although he was moving his arm in the same motion, the difference was truly dramatic. My closest comparison is the softness I feel in my daughter's arm after she's fallen asleep. Yet there was a distinct feeling of firmness coming from deep within his body, and not from his arm. No matter how hard I pushed on his arm, he kept on moving it as if I weren't there. He was able to allow his chi to move me because his muscles were relaxed. Not a lesson goes by in which Master Xu doesn't demonstrate to me the power of relaxation.

A spiritual teacher once gave me a great definition of relaxation. He said, "Relaxation is the absence of unnecessary effort." That sounds simple enough, but it's easier said than done. I began to constantly work with the idea, and when I applied it to my running, it went something like this; the more I could relax my legs and not "effort" with them, the less resistance they created to my forward momentum. It worked so well for me in my races that I was able to run some of the steeper hills in the later miles that I normally would have to walk. The more I play with this idea, the less and less I use my legs as my main motive force, and the more I relax.

The ChiRunning technique allows you to reduce your leg effort, which means to shift the emphasis away from your legs—to get them out of the way so your body can run more easily. It doesn't mean that there's *no* effort, just no *unnecessary* effort. This creates less resistance to your forward momentum. The faster I run, the more I can feel myself move from my center, and the less I need to use my legs. Likewise, the more I gather to my center, the less I use my legs, and the faster I run. The cycle works either way.

Here are some additional benefits to relaxing your muscles. When you are using only your muscles to move your body, you are doing so with a finite amount of energy stored in your muscles. But when you use chi energy to move, you are essentially turning your body into a hybrid machine that operates on two kinds of fuel. It's similar to the hybrid cars that run on gas *and* electricity. The gas engine runs only when necessary (up hills or at higher speeds), and the electric engine takes care of the rest. Similarly, the ChiRunning technique allows you to run with very low muscle usage (gas) because your chi energy (electricity) is doing most of the work. The better you get at accessing your chi, the less muscle fuel you will consume. It doesn't mean you'll never get tired, but it does mean you'll be moving in such an energy-efficient way that your storehouse of muscular energy will take *much* longer to deplete. Can you imagine what your running would feel like if you ran *mostly* on chi?

Here's a letter from a 25-year-old client, Patricia, who recently ran her first marathon in Honolulu after going through the Team in Training Program: "I will do this again. Because of the classes with you I came through this with no hip, knee, or ankle pain. . . . I felt that I could have run another marathon the next day."

Another advantage to being relaxed is that when your muscles are loose and relaxed, the oxygen carried by your blood can enter the muscle cells much more easily than if your muscles are tense. Softer muscles are more absorbent muscles. Just keep telling your muscles, "Softer is better!"

I've been using the theme of Relaxation to learn to run more effortlessly and, also to see how it applies to the rest of my life as well. So far it seems to apply in every situation. As long as I stay relaxed and centered, I more easily accomplish any job set before me—whether it's running a 10K, cooking a meal, or commuting in rush-hour traffic. It seems so much easier to do anything when you offer no resistance to doing it, especially when it's something that you don't like to do! If my legs offer no resistance, the run happens as it should. If I offer no resistance, my life happens as it should.

When you resist or create unnecessary effort or tension in your life, it restricts your flow of energy. A friend of mine who is a body/mind therapist calls this a "nonfreedom." "When someone is internally free," he says, "they move through life with less of the mental tension, worries, uptightness, and fears that are common to us all."

There are about as many ways to be uptight as there are people on this planet. Fears and tension keep us from being ourselves and, more important, from *feeling* ourselves; and they can keep us from running freely. Relaxation creates a sense of freedom in everything, whether it's running, giving a presentation to a prospective client, or handling a child's tantrum. No one can argue with the benefits of being deeply relaxed and focused.

Running is a place where you can begin to explore the potential freedom of deeply relaxing your body. True relaxation comes from possessing a strong center and letting go of all else. ChiRunning offers you the tools to have that strong center while relaxing at the same time.

By the way . . . how did you do with holding your posture?

Exercise

This exercise is intended to be done when you're not running, so you can get the feel of it and then transfer it into your running when you need to. (You'll find that you're also developing your Focusing and Body Sensing skills as you practice this exercise.)

Sit in a chair, lie on the floor, or stand upright. Now inhale and try to tense every muscle in your body at the same time. Hold this pose for a 10-count, then let out your breath and release all of the tension you've been holding. Practice this until you feel like you can release every tight muscle in your body. Be very thorough in tensing every muscle, and be equally thorough in relaxing every muscle. The next step is to do the relaxing part while you're running, and you'll have a great tool to use whenever you need it.

Can you imagine what our world would be like if the four Chi-Skills—Focusing, Body Sensing, Breathing, and Relaxing—were required curricula in all our public schools? These four areas of human experience are, in my mind, such a primary part of our existence that we should all have them as a birthright. We do have these focuses going at different times, but can you imagine having them all engaged at once? The depth of your experience during any activity would be quite different. By practicing these skills in your running, you will eventually find yourself using them in your everyday life, enriching your experience of self and the world around you.

CHAPTER FOUR

The Basic Components of Technique

Spirit needs matter to become substantial; matter needs spirit to become meaningful.—UNKNOWN

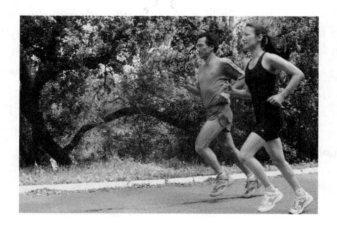

Before we get started on the form focuses, I want to put a carrot in front of you to get you inspired. On your way to truly running by directing your chi, you'll pass through the stage of development I'm about to describe, and this chapter contains the step-by-step process by which you can reach this stage.

Any of these form focuses can, by itself, have a positive effect on your running. But when you can work all of them together and master them, you will be running almost entirely from the pull of gravity, the twist of your spine, and your chi—period.

The essence of this stage in ChiRunning is maintaining a strong centerline in your body, which, when leaning forward, is pulled by gravity. That centerline, remember, runs from the top of your head all the way down your spine to the bottom of your tailbone, and continues down to your point of contact with the ground, your feet. Your hips and your shoulders rotate around that centerline, allowing your feet to keep up with the pull of gravity. What moves your legs is the recoil action of your ligaments and tendons from the twist along your spine, which is a product of your body's natural counter-rotation of the hips and shoulders. What I have just described creates enough energy and momentum for you to run at *your current level*, with what I would safely guess to be *30% of your current energy output.*

When you're standing still, your shoulders, spine, and hips are held in position by all of the ligaments and tendons surrounding them. Running creates a counter-rotation between your hips and shoulders, causing your spine to gently twist. This twisting motion pulls on the ligaments and tendons in your shoulders, spine, and hips, which in turn act like rubber bands wanting to return your spinal twist to its neutral position. With this rubber-band effect, your arms and legs are moving because of the stretch and recoil of your tendons and ligaments, not the contraction of your muscles. The result of this nonmuscular action is greatly reduced perceived effort level, because it is incredibly energy-efficient. Your ligaments and tendons do not require oxygen or glycogen, so less lactic acid is produced when you run. Since your muscles are not being broken down, there is less recovery time needed; and as you run, your joints and ligaments become stronger, more flexible, and healthier. Gravity is pulling you forward, and all of this movement in your body is a response to your forward fall. This technique is how I have been able to do well in ultramarathons on relatively low-mileage training weeks (30 miles per week). Nowadays I spend most of my time working on my technique, and very little time strengthening my leg muscles.

If this doesn't make any sense to you, don't worry. I just want to give you a long-range glimpse of what you have to look forward to.

THE TECHNIQUE

Here we officially shift into the physical aspects of ChiRunning. So far we have talked about the principles of ChiRunning and the Chi-Skills. Now we'll talk about the form focuses. To get an overview of how all this fits together, think of the ChiRunning system as a carriage with the owner riding inside. A driver is sitting on top of this carriage, guiding a well-trained team of horses pulling the carriage down a path toward the next village. The team of horses (the form focuses) is working together as a unit, pulling the carriage (your body) along the path (your running program). They are guided by the driver (the Chi-Skills), who in turn is directed by the owner (the principles).

What does all this add up to? You can have the best carriage in the world, and the most skilled driver, and maybe a very clear vision of where you're going. But if you don't have your horses, you ain't goin' nowhere, partner. And if they're not operating as a team, they'll be working harder than they need to, meaning that you could be in for a long, rough ride. It all comes down to knowing and using the form focuses.

Setting up your running form properly is the first and most important step in ChiRunning. In the beginning you will use more core-muscle effort than you're used to. You might even feel some soreness in your abdominals and hip flexors. This is a sign that you're running correctly and building the necessary support muscles. Over time your body will adjust to this new muscle usage, and as your core muscles strengthen, the effort will no longer seem as great. As your biomechanics improve and your body becomes more energy-efficient, you will actually be able to generate energy as you run, not deplete it.

Even though toning your core muscles takes time, your efficiency will increase right away. Here's a letter from Terry, age 35, a student who attended my beginning level ChiRunning class:

Hi Danny,

I took your three-session class back in July. After the second session, I ran in the San Francisco half-marathon and set a PR [personal record] by taking 9 minutes off my previous best time. Over the rest of the summer I recovered from some minor knee pain, and I've been able to stop wearing the knee support straps I'd been using. At the end of October, I entered the Silicon Valley marathon. Using the techniques I gained from your class, I was able to run the entire race without taking walking breaks, and I completed the distance, taking a whopping 40 minutes off my previous best time!

Terry went into his marathon with a plan of what he wanted to do (the overview of the carriage owner) and what Chi-Skills (the driver of the coach) he would need to run a good race. But none of his dreams would have come to fruition had it not been for his ability to apply good technique (the horses) to running his race.

Changing your running form—or, in some cases, starting from scratch—is a big endeavor. Here are some tips that can make the learning process much more enjoyable.

- **Start simple.** Remember the principle of Gradual Progress: The best things take patience and perseverance. Give yourself lots of time and space to learn this stuff; don't try to take on too much at first. Go slowly and celebrate your small successes. Do only as much as you can do well, and don't worry about the rest—it'll come. Practice the focuses that you're most drawn to, or that you feel will contribute the most to your present condition. (For example, if your posture needs some work, you may want to spend your first few runs focusing on keeping your Column straight.) When you feel comfortable with one focus, add another. Always try to get a clear Body Sense of what you are focusing on before you try to add more. You'll be practicing the principle of Gradual Progress by taking small steps and letting your knowledge grow in a steady and solid way.
- **Have a clear image of what you're supposed to do.** Read and reread the specific focus you're working on until you have a clear understanding of the concept and what you will be doing when you go out to run. If it's a focus that you can practice indoors, by all means do it a few times before you head out the door. The more thorough you are in the beginning stages, the better your chances are of developing a beautiful, smooth running form.
- **Consistency: teach an old dog new tricks.** Your body, like the old dog, learns best with repetition. Learning new habits of movement takes consistency and persistence, and the more often you

practice the form focuses, the more quickly your body will learn them.

I suggest a minimum running program of 3 days a week to start. When you're building a body memory, it's best not to wait too long between practice sessions, because that saves you from having to start from scratch each time you go out.

- **Get a second opinion.** It is sometimes hard to tell if you're moving correctly. One way to solve this problem is to learn ChiRunning with a running partner. If both of you are learning the focuses together, you can act as each other's "eyes" and offer observations of or suggestions on what you see.

Another suggestion is to have your running videotaped so you can see if you're really doing what you think you're doing. The ideal place to do this is at your local high school track. Run the curved section at one end of the track while a friend films you from the infield. This is a great training aid, because it allows you to see a side view of your running form. Borrow a camera if you have to—it's worth it.

A third option is to look at your reflection when you run past a large glass storefront window. Just don't get caught fixing your hair.

Observing yourself offers you the opportunity to practice the ChiRunning principle of Nonidentification. When I first mention in my classes that I'm going to film everyone running, there are always a few groans. But once the students see themselves running, all their worries are replaced with a sense of clarity. When you're not identified, there is no self-judgment going on; you are merely collecting data that will help you to improve your running.

LEARNING THE CHIRUNNING TECHNIQUE: THE FOUR-STEP PROCESS

The basics of the ChiRunning technique are divided into four areas for simplicity. When you have reviewed and practiced the form focuses in each area, you'll have all the basic tools needed to run using the ChiRunning technique. Take plenty of time with these three sections. I suggest that you read and practice all of the focuses in Section I before moving on to Section II, and so on. In Section IV, you'll get out running.

(I) Posture
(II) Lean
(III) Legs and arms
(IV) Let's go running

POSTURE

I begin every run thinking of my posture, so it is naturally the first thing I talk about in my classes. Having good posture is the cornerstone of the ChiRunning technique, and it's crucial to building strong core muscles. When your posture is correct, energy, or chi, flows through your body unhindered, in much the same way that water will flow through a straight pipe more easily than a bent one. Running with your posture out of alignment can create tension, fatigue, discomfort, and even pain. When your posture is aligned properly, your structure is supporting the weight of your body instead of your muscles having to do it.

The principle of Cotton and Steel also applies to posture. Your aligned body has a centerline or axis that runs from head to foot. When your centerline is aligned and strong, it is the "steel" that supports your body, which then allows your arms and legs to relax and become like cotton.

Many people tend to think that posture applies mostly to the trunk. When asked to stand up straight, they don't think about what their legs are doing; they simply adjust their *upper* body. But your *lower* body is equally important. Use the three components below to ensure that you are covering all of the aspects of good posture.

Posture Exercises: Building Your Column
(1) Upper Body Alignment
(2) Lower Body Alignment
(3) Pelvic Tilt

UPPER BODY ALIGNMENT

Exercise

- Start by standing with your feet parallel and hip width apart. Look down to make sure your feet are truly parallel and not turned out. Soften your knees so they're not locked.

- Your trunk: Straighten your upper spine by placing one hand over your belly button and one hand just under your collarbone (figure 6). Pull up with the top hand while pulling down with the other. This will straighten your spine without throwing your shoulders back. Straightening your upper back also opens up your chest cavity, allowing you to breathe more fully and easily.

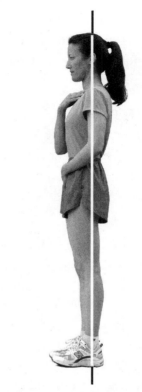

Figure 6—Hands helping posture

- Your head: With the thumb and middle finger of one hand positioned just under your collarbone, let your chin rest on the tip of your pointer finger (figure 7). This will put your head in the correct position—not too high and not too low—and align your neck with your spine. Some runners tend to tip their head back a little when they run, which makes leaning forward (covered below) less efficient and more difficult.

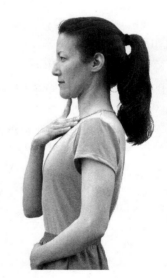

**Figure 7—
The tripod for head position**

LOWER BODY ALIGNMENT

It is important to keep your feet parallel when you practice your posture stance, and even more important when you run. If one or both of your feet turn out when you run, there is a risk of knee injury. As your body moves forward in a straight line, and your foot lands pointing *out* instead of *forward*, it will create a torque on your knee.

Exercise

To correct foot turnout: Rotate your leg(s) in and point your toes forward as you run or walk. Pretend you're running on a tightrope, with the inside of your foot lining up with the centerline of the imaginary rope. Your toes should be pointing in the same direction as your knees (figures 8–11).

With each step, you'll be building stronger adductor muscles, and eventually your feet won't turn out while you're running. When that time comes, all pronation-related injuries could become a thing of the past.

I was a pronator and had chronic knee pain whenever I ran beyond 20 miles. I cured it with these simple focuses practiced on a daily basis. When I'm tired, I still need to remind myself to rotate my knees in when walking or running.

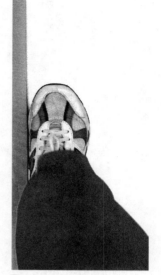

Figure 8—Correct knee/foot alignment

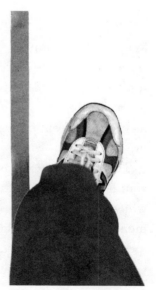

Figure 9—Pronation: incorrect knee/foot alignment

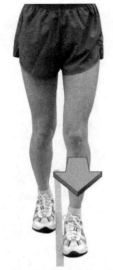

Figure 10—Correct leg/foot alignment

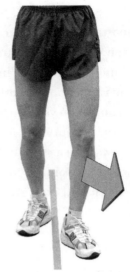

Figure 11—Pronation: incorrect leg/foot alignment

CONNECT THE DOTS
Keep your Column straight, visualize a straight line connecting your shoulder, hip bone, and ankle. Body Sense the base of your Column by feeling your feet on the ground (figure 12).

The following exercise will bring your legs to a truly vertical position, which brings your hips into alignment with your shoulders and ankles, creating the straight line of your Column.

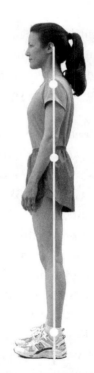

Figure 12—Proper alignment of shoulder, hip, and ankle

Exercise

Once you've straightened your upper body, look down to your feet. If you can see your shoelaces, it's a good bet that your dots are connected in a straight line (figure 13). If you *can't* see your shoelaces, your hips are too far forward (figure 14). Correct this by placing your fingertips on your hip bones and pushing your hips to the rear while keeping your upper body directly over your feet. Once you can see your shoelaces, slowly lift your head up so your eyes are looking straight ahead. Don't move the rest of your body, lift just your head.

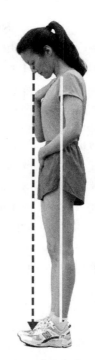

Figure 13—Look down at your shoelaces (correct)

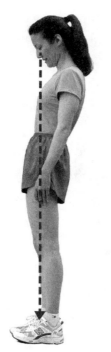

Figure 14—Hips too far forward (incorrect)

If you're used to standing with your abdominals *relaxed* and your hips forward, this adjustment might make you might feel like you're bent at the waist with your butt sticking out. Just look in a mirror to see if you are bent over, or ask a friend to take a look at you. Even though it might feel like you're bent over at the waist, your friend will most likely tell you that you're straight as an arrow.

PELVIC TILT

Master Xu uses the metaphor of the pelvis being like a bowl. If the bowl is tipped forward, it will spill. If it's level, it can hold the contents without spilling (figure 15). If the contents of the bowl represent your chi, then as you tip your pelvis, you spill your chi (figure 16). Keeping your pelvis level does two things: It builds strong core muscles (lower abdominals), and it brings your focus to your center, where your true power lies, allowing you to "contain" your chi.

If your bowl is tipped (a swayed back), much of your core strength will be unavailable, because your core muscles will remain unused or underdeveloped. To avoid tipping your bowl, you'll need to strengthen your abs while relaxing your lower back muscles. Too much curvature in your lower back means your abdominal muscles are overextended and your lower back muscles are too contracted. As you create more of a balance between the front and back sides of your body, there will be more spaciousness in your vertebrae and thus less chance for injury or lower back pain. *Some* curve in your lower back is healthy. Too much curvature can compress the discs in your spine and create pressure on your spinal cord. This can *seriously* cramp your style. I've been there.

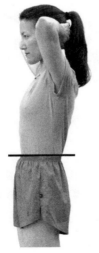

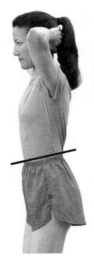

Figure 15—Pelvis level: containing chi

Figure 16—Pelvis tilted: spilling chi

Exercise

Stand upright and lift up your pubic bone with your lower abdominals. *Don't clench your glutes* while doing this exercise. Just isolate and work your lower abs. Each time you pick up your pelvis, hold it for 10 seconds, and then relax. Do this exercise 5 to 10 times a day.

This will help level your pelvis and flatten your lower back. It's a great exercise for those of you with lower back problems, because it strengthens your abs while relaxing your back muscles. It's called flattening your pelvic floor. Do this exercise anytime you find yourself standing on your feet. The more often you remember to do it, the sooner your lower abdominal muscles will get strong enough to hold your pelvis in the right position. Add this focus to the previous one of looking for your shoelaces.

Exercise

If you have an anterior pelvic tilt, commonly known as a swayback, this alternate exercise will help you strengthen your abdominal muscles and level your pelvis.

- Lie on your back with your knees bent and your heels touching your butt.
- Press your lower back into the floor so there is no gap between your spine and the floor.
- Now let your legs slowly straighten as your feet walk away from your lower back. Keep your spine in contact with the earth until your legs are completely straight and your calves are touching the ground. Hold your spine against the ground for as long as you can. This exercise allows you to feel your lower abdominals at work and gives you a distinct feeling of holding your pelvis up while lying in a prone position. It also works to lengthen tight hip flexors. Repeat this exercise 5 times, holding your spine against the ground for 10 seconds each time. Let your calves go only as far down as they can without your lower back losing contact with the floor. When you've reached your maximum, take a deep breath, relax your hips, and let your legs straighten more. Finish by walking your feet back up to the starting position.

IN REVIEW

Here are the three steps to setting up your Column:

(1) Upper Body Alignment: Straighten your upper body with your hands.

(2) Lower Body Alignment: Look for your shoelaces and make any necessary adjustments to your hips.

(3) Pelvic Alignment: Lift your pelvis up in front, using your lower abs, *not* your glutes.

The two key points to Body Sense are your Column, and your feet supporting the bottom of that column. Many people, when taught how to stand with good posture, find it a foreign sensation, because their legs are truly vertical for the first time. When you're standing with correct posture, you will probably feel your abdominals working to hold your Column straight.

I would say that 80% of the runners to whom I've taught these posture exercises started off by standing with their hips too far forward and their legs sloped; their core muscles weren't engaged. Body Sense having a straight Column and memorize what that feels like. Take a mental snapshot and carry it with you, especially when you're running.

The beauty of working to develop good posture is that you can do it anywhere and anytime you feel the urge. Work on your posture whenever you find yourself standing—in line at the grocery store or the bank, or talking with friends at a party. Nobody has to know.

LEAN: GRAVITY-ASSISTED RUNNING

I use the word "lean" to get runners to engage the forward pull of gravity. It is a common mistake to equate leaning with bending forward at the waist (which is very hard on your lower back muscles). When you think of leaning, see it as a full-body tilt in which you fall forward from your ankles instead of bending at the waist (figure 17). Just think of Nordic ski jumpers. Now, *they* know how to lean!

The main reason leaning plays a big role in the ChiRunning technique is because it puts gravity in your favor. Leaning allows gravity

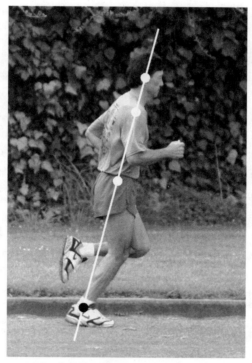

Figure 17—The full-body tilt: leaning from your ankles

to *pull* you forward, instead of your legs having to *push* you, which we all know can be tiring. Here's the scientific explanation: When you stand upright, gravity is pulling straight down on your body along your centerline. As soon as you allow your body to fall forward, your center of gravity moves in front of your point of contact with the ground. This engages gravity to pull you in more of a horizontal forward direction. (I love having gravity do the work.)

YOUR LEAN IS YOUR GAS PEDAL

This is another important attribute of leaning. Your lean is your "gas pedal." If you want to go faster, you simply lean more, and if you want to run slower, you lean less. As you increase your lean, your abdominals work to keep your Column straight and tilted forward. This increase in lean allows gravity to pull you forward at a faster rate, and voilà—your speed is no longer dictated by your leg strength but by your abdominal (core muscle) strength.

FOOT STRIKE: ARE YOU RUNNING WITH THE BRAKES ON?

An additional benefit of leaning is that tilting forward changes where and how your feet strike the ground. Running with a vertical torso— as in power running—makes you reach forward with one leg while you push off with the other. This causes your foot to land in front of you as it hits the ground, which means you're essentially putting on the brakes with every stride. Your knee then becomes the transfer point between the force of your body moving forward and your foot, which is stopping. That's a lot of pressure put on a joint that is not designed to withstand a huge amount of repetitive impact (estimated to be up to six times your body weight with each step!). Knee injuries are by far the most common and the most debilitating of running injuries.

By tilting your body forward from your feet (not from your waist), you place your center of gravity *ahead* of your foot strike. Any physicist will tell you that when this occurs, you are no longer braking, because your feet are moving toward the rear when they strike the ground. This changes your foot strike to the midfoot and allows your legs to *extend* as your feet leave the ground, radically reducing the amount of impact on your knees and quads. As soon as your feet hit the ground, they're gone . . . out the back . . . and there's no braking.

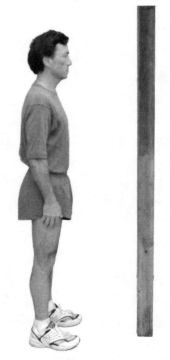

Exercise: Learning How to Lean

- Find a wall to lean against. If you're outdoors and can't find a wall, use anything that will give you rigid support at about waist height—a tree, a fence, a car. Stand facing the wall, with your toes about one shoe

Figure 18—Begin with your posture stance

length away from the bottom of the wall. Find your Column. Pay very close attention to keeping your Column straight *at all times* by engaging your lower abdominals. Hold your hands out in front of you to catch your fall (figure 18).

- Next place your attention on your feet, at the bottom of your Column. Whether you're standing or running, your feet will support your Column whenever they are in contact with the ground. When you relax your lower legs, you'll fall forward and catch your fall with your hands hitting the wall. As you fall

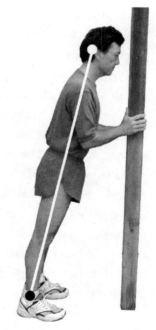

Figure 19—Maintain straight posture while leaning

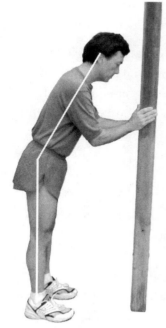

Figure 20—Don't bend at the waist

forward, be sure to keep your Column straight and your ankles relaxed (figure 19). If you're truly relaxing your ankles, your heels won't come off the ground when your body tilts forward. It should feel like your shoes are screwed to the earth. In fact, if you're leaning correctly, you won't even feel an increase in pressure under the balls of your feet. Use that image of the Nordic ski jumper leaning over the tips of his skis. If you bend at the waist when leaning, you'll overwork your lower back muscles (figure 20). Also, don't pull your head

up when you lean, or you'll
weaken your abdominal muscles (figure 21).

- Push yourself back upright and
fall forward again. Repeat this
exercise for 5 minutes: heels
down, Column straight, pelvis
level, ankles and calves relaxed.

- As you repeat this leaning exercise, you should memorize two
sensations (take a physical snapshot):

    1. What it feels like to keep
        your Column straight

    2. What it feels like to have
        that Column falling for-
        ward, pulled by gravity

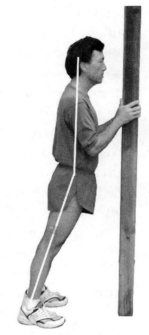

**Figure 21—Posture bent the
wrong way: weak abdominals**

- Stand with your feet together,
and alternate this leaning exercise with all of your weight on
one leg, then the other. After all, when you're running, you land on
only one leg at a time, unless you're some kind of rabbit. Now repeat this exercise until you can do it without breaking the line of
your Column or bringing your heels up off the floor. **Important:**
When you lean forward, use your lower abdominals to hold your
posture straight, NOT your glutes. Clenching your glutes will restrict your leg swing.

Here's an exercise for those of you who want additional practice
leaning and stronger lower-abdominal muscles.

Exercise: Build Abdominal Strength Without Moving a Muscle

Find a table or a park bench which you can lean against with your
quads while letting your body tilt forward (see figure 22). Hold yourself in a straight line while maintaining a lean, and you'll get a great
abdominal workout without moving a muscle! If you want to kill

three birds with one stone you can lay out the morning paper and eat your breakfast this way.

When you do supplemental strength training, it's always best to build your muscles in the motion they will be used. This exercise trains your abdominal muscles to hold your posture straight while tilting forward.

Visualization: Use this great image to help you lean when you're running. Pick a point ahead of you and focus your gaze on it. Then pretend there's a bungee cord running from the middle of your chest to whatever point you picked, and let the bungee cord pull you forward. Don't take your eyes off the point you're focusing on.

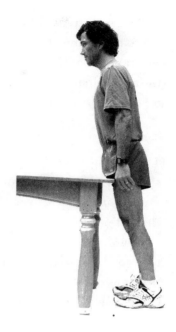

Figure 22—Lean against a table, keeping your posture straight

LEGS AND ARMS

This section is all about getting your arms and legs to let go and move as they should, as an extension of your core, instead of creating an impediment to its movement.

LOWER BODY FORM FOCUSES

This might sound completely counterintuitive, but the faster I run, the less I use my legs. This follows the principle of Cotton and Steel, because the more I lean and use my core muscles (my steel), the more I need to relax and make cotton out of my arms and legs. Triathletes love the ChiRunning technique because after they finish the biking section, they don't have to depend as much on their leg strength to get them to the finish line.

We are all so used to using our legs as the main force in running that to take some of this emphasis away represents a shift in dependence from a familiar muscle group (the legs) to a less familiar group (the abdominals). The following form focuses will free your legs from some of their responsibility.

(1) Pick Up Your Feet

Try this exercise before you read further. It'll take only a second.

Stand up tall with your best posture and let yourself fall forward. That's it.

What happened? Well, if you're like 100% of the other folks who have done this exercise, you let yourself fall forward, just as I asked. As you fell forward, you took a step to keep from falling on your face. There was no push involved with your other leg. In an exercise in Chapter 1, you alternated running in place with picking up your feet. Do you recall how much easier it was to pick up your feet than it was to push your body into the air?

Pushing off with your toes creates too much up-and-down motion and overworks your lower legs, a main cause of shin splints. Picking up your feet allows your body to run smoothly without bouncing. This will ensure that you're moving horizontally forward toward your goal, instead of bouncing along like you're on a pogo stick, fighting gravity with each step.

When you pick up your feet, you'll avoid many common injuries, including shin splints, plantar fasciitis, and knee injuries. You'll also avoid everyone's most feared accident—tripping and falling.

Exercise: Stepping Over the Bar

Here's a great exercise for learning how to pick up your feet instead of pushing off. Stand up right now and walk around in a circle, if you have enough room. You'll notice that the balls of your feet press against the ground (or floor) as you walk. That's because you're pushing off with each step.

Next, pretend that you have an imaginary bar sticking out of the inside of each ankle. In order to walk, you have to pick your foot up over this bar, or you'll trip yourself. Now walk around the room, picking your feet up over your imaginary bars. You should feel much lighter on your feet, and the sensation of the balls of your feet pressing against the floor should be significantly less, if not gone altogether. This is because you are picking up your feet instead of pushing off.

You can practice this exercise whenever you're walking, which for most of us is a significant amount each day. Do it often, and you'll have an easier time remembering to pick up your feet while you're running.

(2) Limp Lower Legs

Contrary to popular belief, your calves are not necessary for endurance running. (If you don't believe me, check out the calves on the next Kenyan you see.) Keeping your lower legs limp at all times while running is the most effective way to prevent injuries to the lower leg. Everything below your knee should dangle when your foot is off the ground. This will ensure that it's not being used—or abused, as is generally the case.

Exercise: Let 'em Hang

- Begin by standing on one leg while shaking your other leg like you've got a gum wrapper stuck to the bottom of your foot. This is the feeling you should have as soon as your foot leaves the ground during your running stride.
- On your suspended leg, loosen your calf, relax your ankle, and soften your foot. Your leg should be totally limp.
- Do this several times for each leg until you can totally relax your suspended leg as soon as it leaves the ground.
- This will train you *not* to push off with your toes while running, thus avoiding any serious lower leg injuries, such as tight calves, plantar fasciitis, shin splints, or hammertoes, to name a few of my favorite sideliners.

The best way to make sure you're not pushing off with your toes is to always keep your lower legs limp from the knees down. If you maintain limp calves and ankles, it's impossible to push off with your toes. Try it if you don't believe me. It's almost impossible to damage a relaxed muscle, and if you never use your anterior tibialis (shin muscle), you'll never get shin splints.

Another way to learn how to pick up your feet while running is to do the sandpit exercise described in Chapter 7 (page 171).

(3) Swing Your Legs to the Rear

Every movement in T'ai Chi is balanced by a movement in the opposite direction. The same holds true for ChiRunning. The principle of Balance says that if a part of your body is moving forward, another part of your body must move to the rear to balance it. Since your upper body is tilting forward, your lower body is responsible for the necessary counterbalance. Let your stride open up *behind*

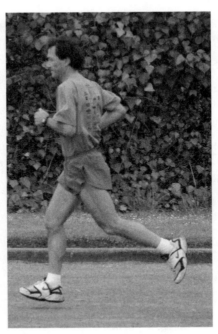

Figure 23—Swing your legs to the rear

you, not in front of you (figure 23). Don't think of swinging your legs forward.

Just relax your hips and let your legs swing out the back. If you reach forward with each stride, your heel will strike in front of you, and you'll be braking with every stride. When your stride opens up behind you, your heels won't strike the ground first, your movement will feel more balanced, and your knees will thank you.

A Visualization: The Wheel

Visualize yourself inside of a big wheel where the top of the wheel (your head) is moving forward, and the bottom of the wheel (your foot) is moving to the rear as you roll down the road (figure 24).

You can also visualize your feet moving in circular patterns, like wheels under you. In figure 17 (see page 71), you'll notice that the "wheels" of your feet are positioned slightly behind your body, unlike a bicycle, where the pedals are under your body.

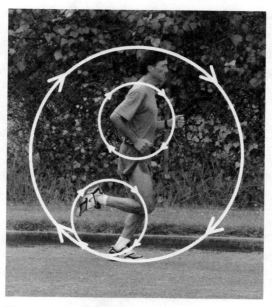

Figure 24—Body Wheels

(4) Loosen Your Hips

As I've said before, the flow of chi through the body is dependent on loose joints. In running, the pelvic area is the center of movement. The legs are swinging in their hip sockets, the pelvis is rotating, and the sacrum and lower back are twisting and swinging along with the pelvis. There are lots of joints moving all at once, and any stiffness in the pelvic area restricts the movement of the entire body. When the pelvis is fully relaxed, you'll have a full range of motion. When running, visualize your pelvic area to be loose and open.

While you're practicing your lean, you'll practice relaxing your lower body and keeping all of your joints very loose. This starts with your lower back. If it's relaxed and loose, your pelvis will swing more easily, which in turn allows your legs to swing fully. Of all the areas of the body that can hold people back in their running, the pelvic area is it. If your hips and lower back are tight, your leg swing will be restricted. Have you ever tried to swing-dance with a stiff back? It doesn't work.

In Chapter 5 there is a section called "Body Loosening Exercises," with exercises showing you how to loosen your joints so your running will be smoother and your chi flowing as it should.

Keeping your hips loose is particularly challenging when you're learning to lean. Intuitively, your glutes and lower back will tense as a survival mechanism brought on by falling forward. Watch for this to happen, and practice relaxing whenever you feel them tensing.

If you do have a stiff lower back or pelvis, ChiRunning will help you loosen the joints that restrict your motion. Just make sure you're always focusing on great posture.

In ChiRunning, it ain't the muscle, it's the motion, and the motion comes from your pelvis and hips.

(5) Cadence

I never paid much attention to my cadence before I started developing the ChiRunning technique. I just figured it was what it was. As I ran faster, my legs turned over faster, which I expected. But once I began to study the physics of efficiency, I realized that I was doing it all backward. Instead of having my cadence go *faster* as I picked up speed, it felt easier to let it stay the same and lengthen my stride as I ran faster. By doing this, my body got used to always running at the same cadence no matter what the speed.

One of the most common and significant problems I see in runners is too long a stride length when running slowly. This is very inefficient and exhausting to the body. If your cadence is slower than 85 strides per minute, your feet stay in contact with the ground longer, which means that your legs are supporting your body weight for a longer period of time. Conversely, if your cadence is over 85 strides per minute, you'll spend significantly less time on your feet, saving valuable energy.

Let's use the example of riding a ten-speed bike to illustrate how cadence applies to your running. Most competitive cyclists try to maintain a pedaling cadence of about 85 to 90 rpm. This allows a steady perceived effort level, no matter which gear they are using. If they want to go faster, they simply keep the same cadence, shift to a higher gear, and speed happens. This combination of cadence with gears also works with running. Your running cadence is measured as the number of strides per minute that each leg takes. Coincidentally, 85 to 90 strides per minute is also a very efficient cadence for runners.

(6) Gears and Stride Length

Everything needs to have gears—cars, bikes, and bodies, too. Utilizing gears in your stride is a great trick that will allow you beginners to run without getting as tired and you seasoned runners to improve your energy efficiency and speed at the same time.

Stride length is to running as gears are to a bicycle. When you're running slowly (in a low gear), you should have a short stride, and when you're running fast (in a higher gear), you'll have a longer stride.

Do the math. A longer stride at the same cadence equals an *increase* in speed. But, your speed increases because you are leaning more and relaxing your legs, not because you are working your legs harder. You don't have to force your stride longer. That will happen naturally as you lean and relax your lower body.

A crucial thing to remember with ChiRunning is that, as you increase your lean, you must also increase the looseness of your pelvis and hips so that your stride can open up *behind* you—not in front of you. This is the opposite of power running, where you open up your stride by lifting your knees and reaching with your legs. This causes your foot to come down too soon, creating too much impact with the ground.

An important point that I would like to emphasize here is how cadence and stride length (or gears) work together to affect your perceived effort level. When these two team up, magic happens. Once you can run at a steady cadence and keep your hips and legs relaxed, your PEL will take on a new dimension, because you are increasing only your use of abdominal muscles, not leg muscles. As you improve your ChiRunning skills, you won't have to think about adjusting your stride length; it will happen naturally, as a function of having relaxed hips and legs. In essence, your legs aren't working harder as you run faster—they're relaxing more.

Gears and Cadence in a Nutshell
- Slower speed = less lean = shorter stride = lower gear
- Higher speed = more lean = longer stride = higher gear
- Tempo always stays at 85 to 90 rpm
- As you lean forward, your stride length opens up out the back

THE METRONOME

The first step in learning to run in different gears is to practice maintaining a steady cadence. I bought a small credit-card-sized electronic metronome at my local music store that works as a great training aid. I'm not big on training gizmos, but this one is simple and produces immediate results. It's really convenient because I can hold it in my hand or stick it in my fanny pack. I set it at 90 and start off running at a slow pace and very short stride length, which gradually lengthens as I lean more. My challenge is to maintain a cadence of 90 whether I'm leaning a little or a lot.

Go out on a run and count the number of steps you take with your right leg over a one-minute period. If it's below 85 per minute, your tempo is too slow, and you're using more leg muscle than you need to.

Practice keeping an even tempo of 85 to 90 steps per minute, no matter how fast or slow you are running. Get yourself a metronome and try it.

UPPER BODY FORM FOCUSES:
WHAT TO DO WITH MY UPPER BODY?

I'm so glad you asked, because in the ChiRunning technique, your upper body contributes a lot.

Think of your body as a team of two, working together to help you run. This "team" consists of your upper body and your lower body, and the more you can get both partners to cooperate and work together, the easier the workload will feel. When you're running on flat terrain, the motion of your whole body should be split between 50% upper body and 50% lower body. There is such an emphasis on the legs nowadays that for many runners these numbers often look more like 10% upper and 90% lower body. When you run either uphill or downhill, these percentages will change. We'll cover that in Chapter 6.

(1) Arm Swing

Here are some suggestions that will help your arm swing.

- **Bend your elbows** at a 90-degree angle and allow your arms to swing from your shoulders in a relaxed way. A bent arm will always swing more easily than a straight arm. Don't pump your arms (opening and closing your 90-degree angle).

  Place your focus on the tips of your elbows, not on your entire arm. It's psychologically much easier to swing a small body part (your elbow) than a large one (your arm).
- **Swing your arms to the *rear*,** not to the front. You're not trying to punch someone in front of you; you're trying to elbow someone behind you. As your body leans forward, swinging your elbows to the rear creates a balance in the opposite direction. The range of mo-

tion of your arm swing should be as follows: Your fingers should come back to your ribs (figure 25), and your elbows should come forward to your ribs (figure 26). If your arms swing forward, it will cause your legs to swing too far forward, creating more heel strike. If you'd really like to swing your arms forward, save it until you're either sprinting or running uphill (see Chapter 7).

- **Keep your shoulders low and relaxed** as you swing your arms. I've met way too many runners who run with tightness in the neck and shoulders from holding the elbows out away from their sides. Letting your elbows pass close to your ribs allows your neck and shoulder muscles to relax.

- **Don't cross your centerline with your hands.** Your forearms will swing slightly across your body, but your hands should not cross your centerline. If they do, it creates too much side-to-side motion in your upper body.

- **Relax your hands.** Hold them with your fingers curled inward and your thumbs on top. Pretend you've just caught a butterfly and you don't want to crush it. (White knuckles are a definite no-no.) Your wrists should be straight and not bent backward. Basically, chi will

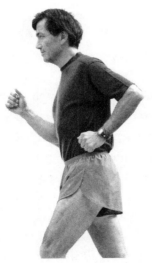

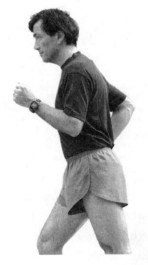

Figure 25—Arm swing: hands to your ribs

Figure 26—Arm swing: elbows to your ribs

not flow through tight joints. And if your joints are tight, your muscles are working more than is necessary.

- **Use your arm swing to set your cadence.** If you're learning to run at 85 strides per minute, set your metronome at 85 beats per minute and swing your arms to the beat. It's so much easier to swing your arms to a beat than your legs, and your legs will automatically swing at the same rate as your arms.

(2) The Pendulum

> It don't mean a thing if it ain't got that swing.
> —DUKE ELLINGTON

Your arms and legs are pendulums. Your arms swing from your shoulders, and your legs swing from your hips. The law of the pendulum states that any pendulum of a given length will always swing at the same rate (swings per minute). If you want a pendulum to swing faster, either you can force it faster, or you can shorten it. If you want your legs to swing faster, there are two ways to achieve that. The first way is to force them to swing faster with your leg muscles, which would obviously increase your muscle usage and fuel consumption. The second way is to *shorten your pendulum* by simply bending your knees. This makes your leg pendulum about half as long as when it is straight, and allows it to swing faster. This is another reason that it's important to pick up your feet: it tricks you into bending your knees.

Try this demonstration of the pendulum effect with your arms:

- Stand upright and let your arms hang at your sides.
- Keeping your elbows locked in this straight position, swing them as fast as you can.
- After about 5 seconds, bend your elbows to a 90-degree angle, but keep them swinging fast for a few seconds and then stop.

Did you feel a noticeable difference in effort when you bent your elbows? Well, the same holds true for your legs: They'll swing more easily if they're bent (figures 27–29).

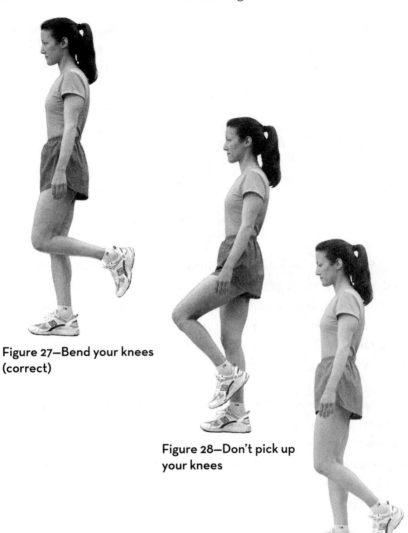

Figure 27—Bend your knees (correct)

Figure 28—Don't pick up your knees

Figure 29—Knees not bent enough

(3) Head, Neck, and Shoulders

Here are a few things worth mentioning about this area of the body.

- **Soften your shoulders.** Since your shoulders are responsible for transferring the motion of your spine to your arms, they must hold as little tension as possible. Try not to use your shoulders to swing your arms. Allow your spine to gently twist and swing your elbows. Everything in between is just a soft conduit for your chi. Use your hat to keep your ears warm, not your shoulders.

- **Keep your neck relaxed** and in line with your spine. Use the three-finger tripod if you're ever in doubt about your head position (see Posture, figure 7, Chapter 4).
- **Look around when you run.** Relax your neck and take in your environment every now and then—there's more to life than trying to remember a gazillion focuses.

LET'S GO RUNNING

Copy these pages and take them with you when you go out to do your first ChiRunning session. I'll talk you through the same sequence that I use in my classes, which has proved itself with the test of time. Let your mind direct your body, and let your body *feel* the focuses. You'll remember each form focus better if you can Body Sense it.

REVIEW OF THE PRERUN FOCUSES
- Begin by practicing your posture stance.
- Stand with your feet parallel.
- Straighten your upper body with your hands.
- Look for your shoelaces.
- Adjust your hips—connect the dots (shoulders, hips, ankles).
- Pick up your head.
- *Feel* your Column from your head to your feet.
- Next, find something to lean against, and do your leaning exercise to remind yourself what it feels like to fall forward.
- Stand 12 inches away from a fence, wall, or tree, facing it.
- Engage your Column.
- Fall forward and push yourself back upright a few times.
- Relax your ankles the entire time.
- Walk around for a few minutes to practice picking up your feet.
- Shake out your legs.

- Maintain your best posture.
- Pick up each foot higher than the opposite ankle.
- There should be no pressure under the ball of your foot as you walk. (Pretend you're sneaking up on someone.)

HOW TO START YOUR RUN

(1) Stand with your best posture and set up your Column.

(2) Bend your arms to 90 degrees and relax your shoulders.

(3) Begin running with a short stride length. Your arms should be swinging gently behind you. (Run slowly enough that your breath rate hardly increases.)

(4) Once you begin running, pretend that you're not running. That's right—imagine you're just practicing your posture stance and that every time your foot touches the ground, it hits at the bottom of your Column, not in front of it. You should feel your midfoot hitting the ground, not your heel. Run this way for a few minutes, and don't think about any other focuses, or even that you're running. It's just you and your Column. Every time your foot comes down at the bottom of your Column, you are connecting the dots (shoulders, hips, ankles).

(5) Run this way until you feel like you can maintain a straight Column (connecting the dots) while running slowly, with a short stride length.

(6) When you feel comfortable holding your Column, drop your attention to your feet and feel how they hit the ground at the bottom of your Column. Now keep your feet hitting at the bottom of your Column while allowing the rest of your Column to tilt forward (*in front* of where your feet are striking). Increase your tilt by only a small amount, and relax into this new angle of lean. Keep your knees down and your lower legs relaxed, picking up each foot over the opposite ankle. This will feel a bit like a prance.

Visualization: This is one of my favorites and always makes my running feel easy. Imagine a bungee cord with one end hooked up to your chest and the other end hooked to an object in the distance. Then, just allow the bungee cord to pull you forward.

Visualization: This will help you remember to pick up your feet. Imagine your feet as two wheels rolling under you, which keep you moving smoothly down the road instead of bouncing up and down wasting energy. If you were running on a treadmill and someone stood beside you to watch your feet, they would see your feet tracing the path of a wheel—very circular. They would see your heels coming up behind you, but they should not see your knees coming up. When you're running and trying to pick up your feet, it's important *not* to pick up your knees, as this will swing your leg too far forward, causing your heel to strike. The phrase to remember here is *Keep your knees low and your heels high.*

Visualization: Pretend that you're pedaling a small bicycle, and instead of pushing down on the pedals, you are pulling up on them.

One of my favorite examples is the Roadrunner cartoon. He has a great lean while his feet are spinning like a wheel behind him.

(7) Hold this new angle of lean for 15 to 30 seconds, then let yourself come back upright. You should feel your speed decrease when you do this. Most people express surprise upon sensing themselves slow down, because they were unaware they had picked up their speed when they increased their lean.

(8) Check in frequently to see that your Column is straight and your feet are still hitting at the bottom of it. Repeat the exercise of increasing your lean and holding it for 15 to 30 seconds, alternating with returning back to an upright position for the same amount of time. Do this leaning exercise 10 times, then take a walking break. When you're leaning, your upper body should be slightly ahead of your foot strike. If it's a race between your head and your feet, your head will always cross the finish line first.

(9) While you're walking, focus on maintaining your Column and relaxing your body.

If your posture is too upright, you will have a tendency to bend at the hips, and your stride will open up in front of your body, creating more impact to your lower back and knees (figures 30–36).

Running with upper body vertical

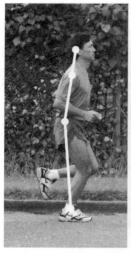

Figure 30

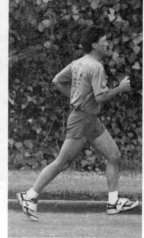

Figure 31

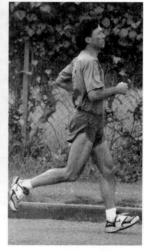

Figure 32

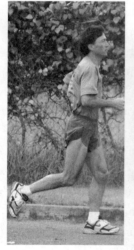

Figure 33

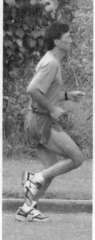

Figure 34

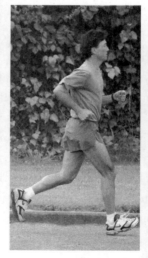

Figure 35

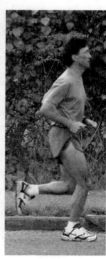

Figure 36

The ChiRunning lean

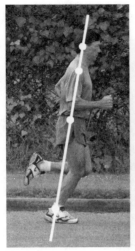

Figure 37

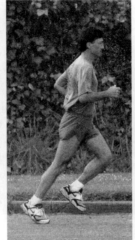

Figure 38

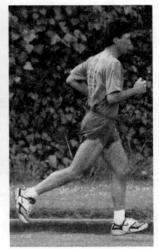

Figure 39

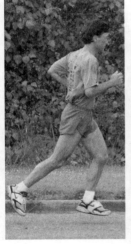

Figure 40

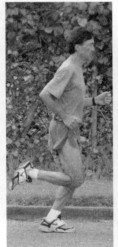

Figure 41

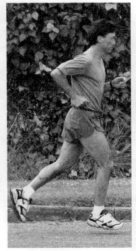

Figure 42

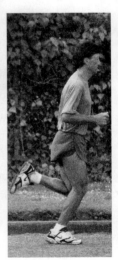

Figure 43

Whereas if your posture is straight and tilted forward from the ground up, then gravity will pull you forward, and your stride will open up behind you, leaving no chance for a heavy heel strike (figures 37–43).

A COMPLETE LIST OF FOCUSES AND REMINDERS

Below is a checklist of all the focuses. Whenever you're practicing a focus, Body Sense it. As you get increasingly proficient with the focuses, you'll be able to sense when some part of your running form doesn't feel quite right, then engage the appropriate focus to correct it.

POSTURE

❑ Straighten your upper body with your hands. Look for your shoelaces.

❑ Keep your legs vertical, not sloped.

❑ Do the "vertical crunch." Lift your pelvis up in front; flatten your lower back slightly.

❑ Tuck your chin and keep your neck in line with your spine. Use the three-finger tripod.

❑ Use the image of a Column—always straight. Connect the dots: shoulders, hips, ankles.

❑ Feel your feet at the bottom of your Column.

LEAN

❑ Keep your Column straight at all times.

❑ Lean from your ankles, with your whole body as one unit.

❑ Feel yourself falling forward.

❑ Be sure your upper body is in front of your foot strike.

❑ Your lean is your gas pedal. To go faster, lean more.

❑ Your upper body is extended out front while your legs swing out the back.

LEGS AND ARMS: LOWER BODY

❑ Pick up your feet.

❑ Keep your lower legs limp.

❑ Swing your legs to the rear.

❑ Bend your knees and let your heels float up behind you.

❑ Remember, soft foot strike, loose ankles, don't push off with your toes. Run quietly and lightly, as if you're trying to sneak up on someone.

❑ Don't pronate. Run along a tightrope, leading with your knees.

❑ Loosen your hips.

❑ Keep your cadence between 85 and 90 strides per minute.

LEGS AND ARMS: UPPER BODY

❑ Swing your elbows to the rear, keeping them bent at a constant right angle.

❑ Don't pump your arms.

❑ Don't cross your centerline with your hands.

❑ Relax your hands, as if you're holding a butterfly.

❑ Keep your shoulders low and relaxed.

❑ Use your arm swing to set your cadence.

GENERAL RUNNING TIPS

This is a quick reference list of focuses to remember when you're starting your runs. The best way to get familiar with the focuses is to pick one or two and work with them until you can clearly Body Sense each one. Then, on a subsequent run, pick two different ones. Work your way through the list, and when you finish, start at the top of the list . . . ad infinitum.

❑ Keep your stride length short as you take off. Let it lengthen gradually as you lean more.

❑ Keep your lower legs limp.

❑ Pick your foot up over your opposite ankle, and don't push off with your toes.

❑ Remember the wheel. Pretend you're pedaling a small bicycle.

❑ Lean from your ankles by tilting your Column forward.

❑ Let your feet hit at the bottom of your Column. Your upper body should always be ahead of your foot strike.

❏ Land midfoot, just behind the balls of your feet, not on your heels.

❏ Swing your arms and legs to the rear.

❏ Let gravity pull you. Use the bungee-cord image.

❏ Keep your shoulders relaxed and low.

❏ Keep your knees down and your heels up.

❏ Look for that gentle twist along your spine. Let your hip be pulled to the rear as your leg extends behind you.

❏ Keep your cadence between 85 and 90 strides per minute.

❏ When you get tired, shorten your stride length and come back up on your lean slightly.

❏ Smile!

Granted, it's a lot to think about . . . but so is a car when you first learn to drive. You don't have to learn this by next week. In fact you have the rest of your life to master these focuses, so don't pressure yourself to learn it all at once. Just take it in small increments one day at a time and you'll be a happy runner.

The ChiRunning form, though important, is only the beginning of learning to run and live from your center. Read on to catch a glimpse of the bigger picture and come back to this chapter when you're ready to run.

CHAPTER FIVE

Transitioning into and out of Running

The beginning holds the seed of all that is to follow.
—I CHING

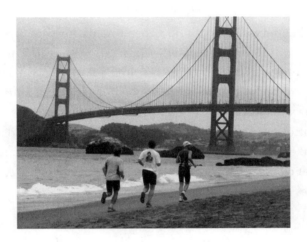

A s much as I stress the importance of good running form, it's the setup and approach that dictate the *quality* of a workout. The most important part of a running program is obviously the running, but I would say that transitioning takes a very close second.

A transition is a conscious pause. It is a time to take stock of yourself and think about the run you are about to begin. The space before a run is like the pause between breaths. It's the thoughtful moment that precedes movement, when you set up your intentions of what you'd like to do during your run. It's your opportunity to ponder what you'd like to focus on, whether it's pacing, focuses, weak areas of form, recovering your legs, scouting new running routes, or just breaking in shoes.

One of my favorite times to watch elite athletes is just before a race.

I imagine them playing the whole scenario of what they're about to do in their heads. They're trying to focus and relax at the same time—and the ones who are most successful at doing both are the ones who are usually at the head of the pack.

Transitioning also includes the time after running, when you relax and review what you just did. Not judging what you did, simply observing it and making note of anything that stands out. There's no such thing as a bad run, no matter how you may feel during or afterward. That's because there's always something of value that you can come away with—always a lesson to be learned, if you're looking for it.

This chapter will tell you how to get ready for your next run, and how to recover from and make the most out of your last run. You will learn the importance of moving into and out of your runs in a mindful way. I will also discuss what you can do between runs to ensure that all of your workouts are high-quality.

Transitioning properly into and out of your runs will not only have beneficial effects on your workouts; it can also be used as an everyday ritual that connects your running with the rest of your life, making it a sacred event, which it is.

TRANSITIONING INTO A RUN

PREPARING YOUR MIND

Moving into your next workout mentally prepared means assessing your present state and considering what you might want to do during the upcoming run. When you're getting ready to go out for a run, the following steps will make your preparation more thorough and your running practice more intentional.

- **Look at the big picture.** What type of run is on the schedule? Is there some aspect of this training run that you should pay particular attention to?
- **Body-sense,** or check in with, yourself—get a clear sense of your present state. Try to feel if there is anything going on in your body that could adversely influence your run, either physical, emotional,

or mental. Various examples could be: illness, fatigue, low energy, injuries, stiff or sore muscles, a full stomach, tension or worry, time constraints, basically anything that could draw you away from having a clean undistracted run.

- **Adjust your run** if you need to accommodate something going on in your body. For example, if you have stiff muscles, you might want to start off a bit slower and let the soreness work its way out before you pick up the speed.

- **Know specifically what you will be doing** so your energy and focus are best utilized during your run. What will your focuses be? What is the most important thing for you to practice on this run? What are your intentions? What would you like to come away with?

- **Watch yourself.** Commit yourself to checking in at regular intervals. I set the countdown timer on my watch to go off every five minutes. The beep serves as an alarm clock bringing me back to my focuses and intentions. This works better than anything I've ever tried. It will take much longer to improve your form if you practice only during the first few minutes and then forget to do it for the remainder of your run.

PREPARING YOUR BODY

How many times have you gone out for a run and felt like your legs were made of concrete or worse? Well, I'll clue you in on a little secret. They might not feel so bad from something you *did* as from something you *didn't* do. Most people don't realize that taking good care of their body *between* runs is the best way to optimize the enjoyment and effectiveness of their workouts.

Here are some steps to take before going out for a run.

- **Eating**

    If you eat before you run, be sure it's at least three hours before. If you run in the morning, it's not really necessary to eat anything before you head out. Almost nothing you eat immediately before a run will be far enough into your system to help you. If you do have to eat before running, be sure it's not a big meal, or you might end up with heartburn, stomachache, side stitches, or leaving it on the road somewhere. I've never heard of anyone starving to death on a run. In fact, if I'm hungry before I go running, it usually subsides within the first mile or two. It's best to run on an empty stomach, even on race days (with the exception of marathon distance or longer). Eating well the night before allows you to get up, get dressed, and head out in the morning. Then the biggest decision you might face is which route to follow.

- **Hydrating**

    If you run regularly, get yourself into the habit of drinking water all day long. It is recommended that the average person consume between 64 and 100 ounces of water daily, depending on a daily caloric expenditure of 2,000 to 3,000 calories. That's ten 10-ounce glasses of liquid. For the sake of your health, I'd suggest that it be mainly water, preferably filtered and not distilled. There are other forms of libation, but they all involve an increase in the work of your kidneys to filter out the extraneous ingredients. To keep from getting dehydrated, drink at least 8 ounces of water a half hour before heading out. If you're going longer than 5 or 6 miles, take along a water bottle or plan a route that has water stops along the way. Staying well hydrated will help your legs avoid cramping and keep your core body temperature within a reasonable range, especially in hot weather.

- **Shoes**

    Make sure your shoes aren't too tight. If they are, you might feel a slight pain in your arches. Your feet can move much more freely when they're not held hostage by tight shoes.

- **Prerun Body Looseners**

    I've never been very big on stretching before runs, out of a healthy fear of pulling a muscle. There is really no need to stretch your muscles if you start off very slowly and warm up your muscles for the first ten minutes of each run.

    Do this set of Body Looseners before you head out the door. I call them "looseners" rather than "stretches" because they're meant to loosen your joints, not stretch your muscles. They're actually warm-up exercises for T'ai Chi, but if you do them religiously before you run, they will work wonders on the fluidity of your stride. If your joints are open and loose, your chi flows through your body unhindered. Also, your muscles don't have to work as hard to flex joints that are loose. One of my longtime students has gotten so much benefit from these exercises that she now refuses to run unless she's done her Looseners first.

This set of exercises is designed to loosen the main joint systems of the body, which are:

- Ankles
- Knees
- Hips
- Sacrum
- Spine
- Shoulders and neck

Body Loosening Exercises

Begin by shaking out your lower legs and then your whole body. Let yourself get really floppy and loose.

- **Ankle rolls:** These will loosen all the ligaments and tendons in and around your ankles.

  Put your toes on the ground just behind your opposite foot. Keeping your toes on the ground, roll your ankle around in circles, letting your knee do the work so that your ankle can relax. Do 10 clockwise circles and then 10 counterclockwise. Switch legs and repeat the exercise.
- **Knee circles:** This motion loosens the ligaments around your knees. Place your hands on your knees and

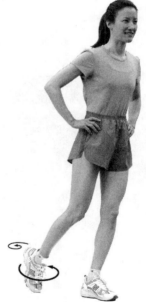

Figure 45—Ankle rolls

move them around in clockwise circles, then reverse the direction. Do 10 in each direction.

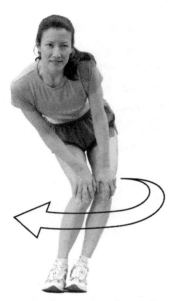

Figure 46—Knee circles—left

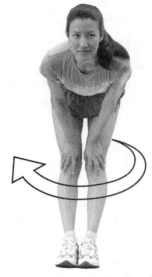

Figure 47—Knee circles—back

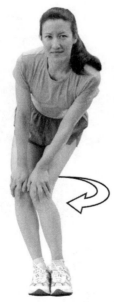

Figure 48—Knee circles—right

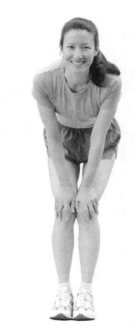

Figure 49—Knee circles—front

- **Hip circles:** This exercise is easy to do but can be challenging to learn. It is, however, one of the best exercises there is for loosening the ligaments and tendons in your hips and pelvic area. Just take it slowly, and it'll come. I'll take you through it one step at a time.

  Stand up straight with your best posture stance. Be sure to keep your knees slightly bent. Relax your hips, and move your right knee in a circular clockwise direction. Your whole foot will be in contact with the ground at all times. Do 5 "practice" circles, then return to your original stance. Do 5 clockwise circles with your left knee. Now do the full exercise with *both* legs moving in a clockwise direction but a half-cycle out of sync with each other (figure 50). If you start by moving your knees very slowly, it will come easier, you can always speed up as you get used to it. Start your knees going in circles by moving your right knee forward and your left knee back. This will get them each moving

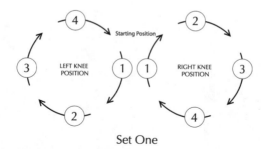

Set One

Figure 50—Hip circles

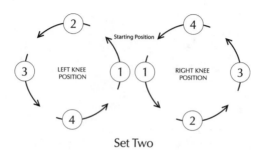

Set Two

Figure 51—Hip circles

in their respective clockwise circles. When they come back around to complete the circles, you will be in your starting position. Switch directions and repeat the exercise. Start with 10 circles in each direction. This exercise can be done anytime and anywhere, whether you're running or standing in line at the theater. It works to loosen your hips and pelvic area which is where the bulk of movement happens in your running. Loosening this area makes your running very fluid and easy.

- **Pelvic circles:** This exercise really works to loosen the area around your sacrum, which plays a key role in allowing you a loose and relaxed leg swing.

    Place your hands on your hips; keep your back and spine in a vertical position; and tip your pelvis forward, to the side, to the back, to the opposite side, then back to forward. Do 10 full circles with your

Pelvic circles

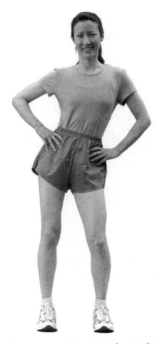

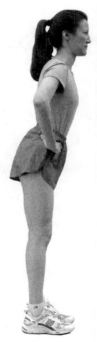

Figure 52—Hips to the right   Figure 53—Hips to the back

pelvis and then change direction. When you get smooth at this one, it will feel like you're belly dancing. Keep your upper body as motionless as possible as you make the circles with your pelvis.

• **Spine rolls:** This exercise works to loosen all the ligaments along your spine.

Stand up straight and bend forward at the waist, keeping your upper body posture straight. When you get as far over as your hamstrings will allow, stretch your spine in both directions by pushing on your hips and craning your neck at the same time. (This will loosen your spine by creating microspaces between each of the vertebrae.) Hold this stretch for 5 seconds, then soften your knees, flop over at the waist, and let your upper body just hang there, upside down. Bend your knees slightly, and starting with your tailbone, straighten yourself up one vertebra at a time until you are vertical again. Do this very slowly. Repeat 3 times.

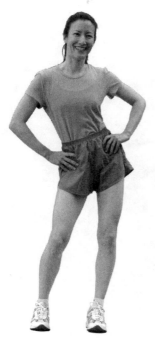

Figure 54—Hips to the left

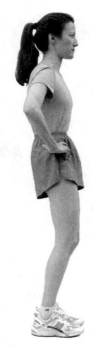

Figure 55—Hips to the front

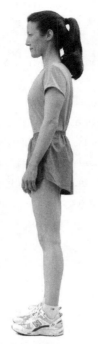

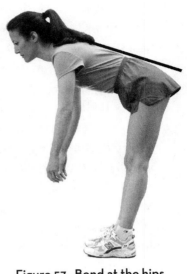

Figure 57—Bend at the hips and keep your back flat

Figure 56—Spine-roll starting position

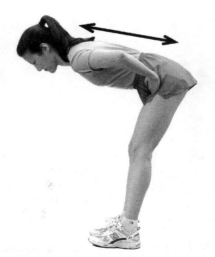

Figure 58—Stretch your spine in both directions

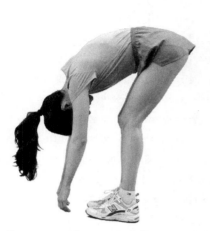

Figure 59—Flop over and hang limp

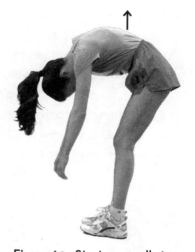

Figure 60—Start your roll at the lower back

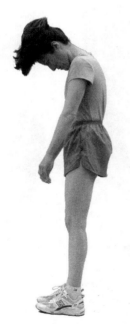

Figure 61—The last thing to lift is your head

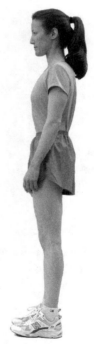

Figure 62—Back to the starting position

- **Spinal twist:** This one works to loosen the ligaments in your upper spine and shoulders, allowing you a relaxed arm swing.

  Stand with your feet together and your posture as upright as you can make it. Interlock your fingers behind your head with your elbows out to the sides. Keeping your hips in a stationary position, rotate your upper body to the right. As you twist your upper body around, drop your right elbow and raise your left elbow so that your upper body is bent to the side. When you're twisted around, look down and try to see your opposite heel. Hold this position for a couple of seconds, then come back to your starting position. Do the same thing on the left side. Repeat this exercise three times.

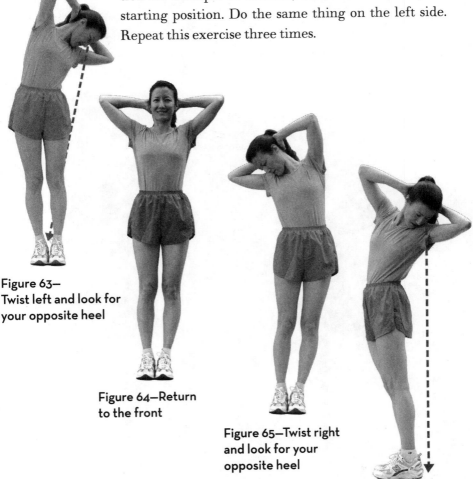

**Figure 63—
Twist left and look for
your opposite heel**

**Figure 64—Return
to the front**

**Figure 65—Twist right
and look for your
opposite heel**

**Figure 66—Side view
showing line of sight**

- **Shoulders and upper back:** Stand with your feet parallel and hip width apart. Then step straight back with one of your feet so the toe of that foot is lined up with the heel of the forward foot (as if you're starting a race), with your forward knee bent and your rear leg straight (figure 67). Your weight should be a little more over the front foot than the rear one. Lean your upper body out over your forward leg, keeping your spine straight. Now let your neck, arms, and shoulders totally relax while rotating your pelvis clockwise, then counterclockwise, in a back-and-forth motion (figure 68). Keep your arms and shoulders completely relaxed, and let them be swung by the rotation of your pelvis. Feel the twisting motion in your lower back. Let your elbows bend

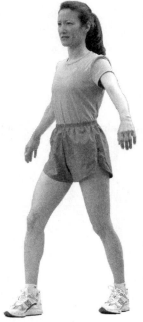

Figure 67—One foot behind the other: front leg bent, rear leg straight

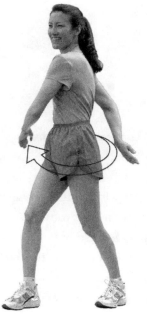

Figure 68—Use your hips to swing your shoulders

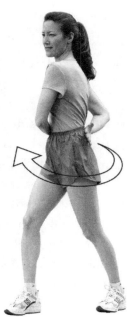

Figure 69—Bend your elbows

as they swing behind your body so that the swinging motion won't pull on your shoulders (figure 69). Now shake out your whole body and finish with the grounding stance.

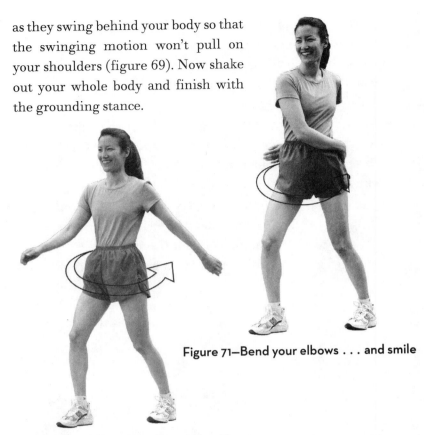

Figure 71—Bend your elbows . . . and smile

Figure 70—Rotate hips in opposite direction

- **Grounding stance:** In ChiRunning, every foot strike is an opportunity to feel your feet on the ground and your structure supported by the earth. Do this exercise before every run to ground yourself in your body and feel the power of the earth beneath your feet.

  Stand upright with your best posture. Place your feet hip width apart and parallel. Soften your knees and let your arms hang at your sides. Feel your posture straight and tall. Focus your attention on your *dan tien* (your center, located three fingers below your navel). At the same time, drop your attention to the bottoms of your feet, and press your big toes softly into the ground. Now connect your *dan tien* to your feet with an imaginary line and let your feet support you. This will have the effect of rooting you to the earth. Hold this for at least 30 seconds. It'll feel like a long time, but it's worth every second if it leaves you feeling grounded. Master Xilin, my first T'ai Chi teacher, had me stand this way for the duration of our $1^1/_2$ hour class—for weeks! He explained that it wouldn't do me any good to try to learn T'ai Chi if I couldn't feel grounded in my body first. Master Xu says it's one of the most difficult stances in T'ai Chi to master. I'm still working on it.

If you have access to one of those large stability balls, here's a great exercise to help get your body in the right alignment for the grounding stance. I call it the Chi-ball exercise.

(1) Start by holding the ball in front of your body with your arms wrapped around it. Soften your knees and let the weight of your body sink into your feet (figure 72). Take a body snapshot of the position of your body and the physical sensations connected with it.

(2) Now drop the ball while holding your body position (figure 73).

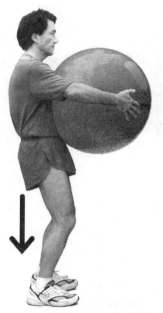
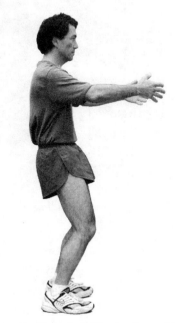

Figure 72—Hold the Chi-ball and sink   Figure 73—Remain in the body position

(3) Next, relax your arms and let them fall to your sides without disturbing your body position. This is the grounding stance (figure 74).

(4) Here's what the grounding stance looks like in motion: Subtract the left leg and tilt the runner upright, and there it is. In ChiRunning, every time your foot hits the ground, that's your grounding stance (figure 75).

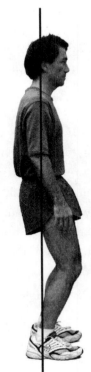

Figure 74—Lower your arms

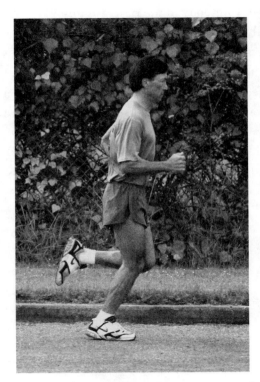

Figure 75—The grounding stance in your stride

After doing the body looseners, check in with yourself by Body Sensing how your body feels in the moment. Are you tense, sore, tired, or stiff? Do you feel pressed for time? Are you grounded? Is there anything you need to consider as you begin your run?

- **Starting your run:** The first thing you should always do before starting a run is your posture stance. Use it to reconnect with the earth and to feel your Column in place. Hold it until you have a clear sense of your Column from head to foot, then shake out your lower legs before you take your first step. Start off at a very easy pace—so easy, in fact, that your breath rate doesn't increase. I'm talking creepy slow, first gear with tiny steps. As you begin to run, relax your body. Keep everything as limp as possible; let your step and cadence gently shake your body. It's a little like a running massage. You're really just shaking your muscles and skeleton to take the edges off. When you feel sufficiently relaxed, start to bring the focuses into your run. The first thing to think about is your posture. Then let your lean enter in, followed by re-laxing your shoulders and swinging your arms. Last, let your feet begin doing the Wheel. After 5 minutes, you'll find yourself run-ning along, loose and happy. As you feel more warmed up, you can increase your pace slowly until you're running comfortably at the speed you'd like. If you start off too fast, you'll use up most of your energy and have nothing left for later. Your goal should be to pace yourself so that, at the end of your run, you are pleasantly tired, not wasted.

  The beginning of your run is a study of Gradual Progress, be-cause you are starting off very small and allowing your body to increasingly relax in its motion. If your run unfolds in this way, you will feel better and better as you progress toward the finish. Then everything will be working in your favor: Your hips will be open and relaxed, your cadence will be steady, your breathing will be settled and regular, your muscles will feel used but not abused, and you'll be feeling more energized than when you started.

TRANSITIONING OUT OF A RUN

You've just finished running. You're feeling pleasantly tired, and it's time to move on to your next activity. This is precisely the time to begin preparing for your next run. Sound crazy? Not so. In order for you to have a good run, whether it's tomorrow or the next day or next week, the best thing you can do for yourself is to "clean out" your legs and treat them to a nice recovery. It's like a gardener cleaning her tools after using them, or a carpenter putting everything back in his toolbox after a day's work. In either instance, when the work is started up again, everything will be in order, and the gardener or carpenter will have a fresh start, with no carryover from the last session. If you take good care of your legs between runs, the quality of your next running session will be greatly enhanced.

Complementary to the prerun themes of preparation and intention, the postrun themes change to recovery and assessment. After a run is the time to allow the results of your efforts to settle into your body and the time to do what it takes to physically recover so you can move into your next activity with a clear mind and a rejuvenated body. The mental aspect involves using your mind to assess how your run went—what you got from it, how it felt, what you learned, what worked and what didn't, and what you might do differently next time. The physical and mental emphases are still there, but in different capacities.

Just as events in Nature are cyclical, your running program will fall into a cycle of preparation, action, recovery, and rest. Use the seasons as your model. Spring is the time of preparation. The seeds that lie in the ground are moistened by the spring runoff. As the air gets warmer, the seeds sprout, and by midsummer they are maturing into full-grown plants, bearing fruit. As the summer rains disperse and the autumn days grow shorter, the fruit falls, leaving seeds that will sprout in the spring. The leaves fall, helping the earth recover nutrients that were used up by the growing plants. Then comes winter, when everything rests under a blanket of snow and darkness, waiting for the spring thaw to start the whole cycle again. It's no different from the cycle of a well-thought-out running program. If the cycle works so well for Nature, why not borrow some of that wisdom for yourself?

One way I remind myself of the seasons' cycles is by celebrating the two solstices and the two equinoxes with my family and friends.

We celebrate each with simple rituals that represent what is happening in Nature at the time.

Whether we know it or not, we all have our own rituals. It could be anything from washing your car to having a cup of warm milk before sleep. I have a very enjoyable ritual for transitioning out of a run that you might like.

- **Ending a run:** After your run is when you can do the most to ensure that your legs will be fresh and ready for the next workout. Don't just jump back in your car and head off to your next event, or you could be walking around with tight legs for the rest of the day. Give yourself a little time to switch out of running and into the rest of your day. A cooldown and stretching period allows excess lactic acid to be flushed into your bloodstream and eliminated from your body. If it is allowed to linger in your system, studies show that it turns to concrete, or worse.
- **Cooling down:** When you cross your imaginary finish line, don't stop running. That's right, don't stop running—but reduce your speed to an effortless jog. This will allow your muscles to stay warm and help to circulate much of the metabolic waste out of your system. Take five minutes to jog at a very relaxed pace before slowing to a walk. Then take a few minutes to Body Sense how you feel. Let the run settle in to your body. You should feel pleasantly tired, not exhausted. Walk until your breath rate drops and your heart rate returns nearer to normal.
- **Stretching:** Even though I don't stretch before I run, I always stretch afterward. Here are a few injury-prevention guidelines for stretching. If you do it right, it will have an uncanny resemblance to yoga.

  Listen carefully to your body. I've seen too many people have great workouts and then pull a muscle while stretching.

  Never stretch a muscle until it hurts. Your stretches will be more effective if you take a soft and gentle approach.

  Relax and breathe out as you initiate each stretch.

  Hold each stretch gently for at least 30 seconds. Body Sensing will tell you how much stretching your body needs and how much it can handle.

(1a) **Calf stretch:** Lean against a wall with one heel extended on the ground behind you and the opposite foot on the ground at the base of the wall in front of you (figure 76). Move your pelvis toward the wall. This will stretch the calf muscles in your rear leg. Hold for a count of 10 and repeat 3 times on each leg.

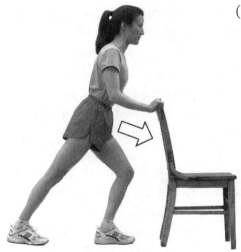

(1b) **Achilles stretch:** Same position, except you are dropping your rear knee down toward your forward heel. Hold for a count of 10 and repeat 3 times on each leg.

(2) **Hip flexor and upper hamstring stretch:** Rest one foot on top of a chair and move your pelvis toward the raised heel. Hold for a count of 10 and repeat 3 times on each leg. Keep your trunk vertical.

Figure 76—Calf/Achilles stretch

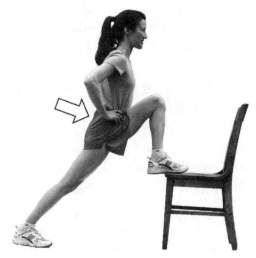

Figure 77—Hip flexor and hamstring stretch

(3a) **Hamstring stretch:** Place one heel on something hip height. Keeping both knees and your spine straight, bend your trunk toward your raised foot. Bend only as far as your hamstrings allow. Hold for a count of 10 and repeat 3 times on each leg.

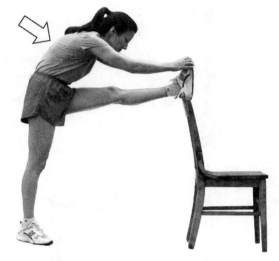

Figure 78—Hamstring stretch

(3b) **Adductor stretch:** Keeping your raised leg in position, turn your body 90 degrees and let your upper foot rest on its side. With your spine straight, bend down to touch the toes of your support legs. This will stretch your adductors. Hold for a count of 10 and repeat 3 times on each leg.

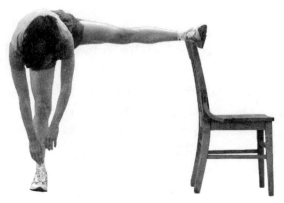

Figure 79—Hamstring/adductor stretch

(4) **Quadriceps stretch:** With your right foot on the ground, grab the ankle of your left leg with your left hand and pull up on your heel. Keep your knees together. Reach straight up over your head with your right hand. This move not only stretches your quads but builds the core muscles required for good balance. If you want to increase the stretch, hold this posture while picking up your pelvis in front. Hold for a count of 10 and repeat 3 times on each leg.

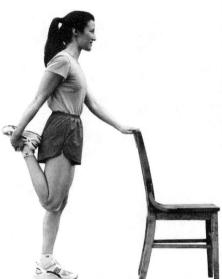

Figure 80—Quadriceps stretch

(5) **Latissimus dorsi (lats) stretch:** This stretches the muscles of your lower back just below your shoulder blades. Stand vertical with your feet widely spread. Hold your arms horizontally out to your sides with your thumbs up. Tilt your upper body to one side until your arms make a vertical line, with one hand down and one hand up. Hold for a count of 10 and repeat twice on each side. In yoga this is the triangle pose.

• **Soaking your body:** If you have the luxury of being able to take a hot bath after your workout, do it. Soaking your legs warms your muscles and relaxes them back into their normal shape. Soaking in hot water dilates your capillaries, which helps to flush metabolic waste out of your muscles and into your bloodstream to be eliminated. A hot shower doesn't work as well, but it's still good for your legs, if a bath is not an option.

There seems to be a huge ongoing debate as to whether heat or cold is better for your legs after running. Cold is recommended if you have any inflammation, because it gets blood to circulate to the injury. But if you're not injured, cold doesn't make any sense, because it causes your muscles to contract, trapping the metabolic waste. After a hot bath, it's fine to do a cold soak. In fact, it feels very refreshing and allows your legs to feel more cohered as you move on to your next activity.

Hot baths have been one of my favorite rituals after running. And given the hectic nature of our fast-paced world, I recommend hot baths whether you run or not.

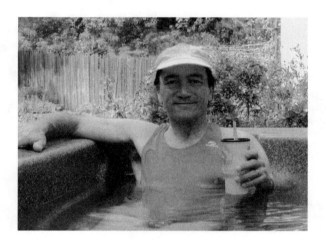

- **Leg drains:** When you're finished with your bath, do some "leg drains" by lying on your back with your feet propped up against a wall for 3 to 4 minutes (figure 82). Close your eyes and relax your entire body for 3 minutes. Then, using your hands, start at your ankles and squeeze down your legs toward your heart as if you're trying to wring the water out of a wet towel. This will allow the blood to drain out of your legs so that fresh clean blood can be pumped back in when you stand up. If your legs are not "cleaned out" after each run, you could start your next run with some of the "exhaust" from previous runs, which is no fun at all.

You can do leg drains either immediately after stretching or after your bath. Either way you'll notice a markedly different pair of legs under you when you get up. This is a great exercise to do any-time your legs feel tired. It's especially good for those of you who work on your feet. All you need is about three square feet of floor space with an adjoining wall, and you can have fresh legs in min-utes. Try it. You'll be amazed.

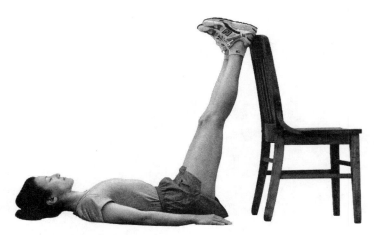

Figure 82—Leg drains

- **Eating after your run:** Even though you might feel hungry right after running, it's best to wait at least 45 minutes to an hour before eating. Let your heart rate, breath rate, and body temperature come back to normal before taking in food. If you wait to eat, you'll be settled and more deeply nourished when you sit down to your next meal.

  If you've just done a strenuous workout, one of your next two meals should contain a good helping of protein, which will give your muscles the necessary building blocks for cellular reconstruc-tion. It's also good to get in a hearty salad, with lots of fresh greens and vegetables, to put valuable minerals back into your system.

- **Rehydrate:** Drink plenty of water after running. The rule that I use is "Drink before you get thirsty." If you finish a run with a dry mouth, your body is letting you know you didn't drink enough.

Keep a steady flow of water going in after your workout, drinking small amounts until you're no longer thirsty. If you're tempted to grab a soft drink, just remember this: Your kidneys are already stressed from doing overtime on the run, so it's a bit unfair to create more work for the poor little things by dumping in a bunch of chemicals and sugar. Stick to water or unsweetened fruit juice, and your kidneys will be happy as clams.

The more time you spend taking care of your body between runs, the more it will reward you with many years of enjoyable workouts. You'll also notice an increase in your performance levels and the quality of your workouts.

THE POSTRUN MIND

- **End-of-run review:** I highly encourage an end-of-run review. The end of a run is another important time to practice Body Sensing and get as much data from your body about your run as possible. Start by simply comparing how you felt at the beginning of the run to how you felt at the end. This data will help you build the best possible running program for your body. It will teach you more about running than twenty books could. Your body will tell you if the run was too long or too fast. If your legs are tired, you'll know you need to practice using limp lower legs next time and per-haps shorten the distance. Specific muscle soreness will tell you where you were inefficient with your form and what to relax next time.

- **Keep a running log/journal:** I suggest keeping a running log, and, if you want to be really thorough, write in a journal.

    Here are a few good reasons to keep a log:

    - You can track your progress as you move through your train-ing program.
    - You can check in with the time schedule of your training pro-gram.
    - You can keep track of injuries to avoid future mistakes in your training.
    - You can log your weekly miles, which is very useful as a topic

of conversation if you're ever caught at a cocktail party with nothing to say. ("Wow, you ran *that* far in a week?")

- You can learn from what isn't working in your running schedule and make appropriate adjustments.
- You can give yourself a nice positive acknowledgment for how far you've come since you started all this craziness.

Things to Track and Journalize

- Daily and weekly mileage
- Average pace on training runs
- Number of intervals and their relative split times (if done on the same course)
- Results of Body Sensing after a workout
- Aches and pains: location and intensity, what you were doing at the time
- Notable breakthroughs in your understanding of how your body is doing with the ChiRunning technique
- The age of your running shoes

CONCLUSION

The key word for transitioning into and out of your running is "mindfulness." Being mindful during the time between runs will allow you to arrive at your current workout recovered and ready to be fully engaged. When you approach your running mindfully, each workout becomes more like a personal ritual. Not a blind ritual, full of form yet lacking substance, but a *living* ritual that leaves you with a sense of intention and depth.

By involving both your mind and body in your transitions, you will learn much more than good running skills. You'll develop qualities of thoughtfulness and presence that you can carry with you into the rest of your life.

The ChiRunning technique is about being respectful to your body while you run. Transitioning is about being respectful to your body between runs. As you practice all of your running and transitioning focuses, a ritual of your own will take shape organically from the cycles of exercise and recovery that you put yourself through in the course of your program.

This approach to your running can help you live a life that is both focused and relaxed—two very useful qualities that *I'd* like to have when I grow up.

CHAPTER SIX

Program Development: The Process of Growth

We are what we repeatedly do. Excellence, then, is not an act, but a habit.—ARISTOTLE

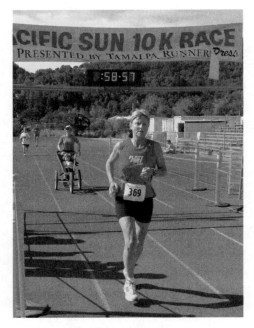

Figure 83—Nancy Weninger, age 55, triathlete and ChiRunning student

Program development adds the ingredient of *duration* to your form focuses. Whether it's measured in minutes for a beginner, or in hours for a marathoner, a part of the process of learning the ChiRunning technique is integrating the form focuses into your running for longer periods of time. This is where having a well-planned running program will guarantee safe and successful development, one based on the core principles of ChiRunning.

The Formula for Success

The formula for developing a successful ChiRunning program is *form, distance, and speed*—in that specific order. This three-stage method will guarantee that your program will build safely and gradually because you won't fall prey to the power running mind-set of "no pain, no gain" and get injured by overtraining.

You will work on your *form* before anything else. As you are able to hold that together for longer periods of time, you will be building core strength while becoming looser and more relaxed. Together, these components create the foundation for increased *distance*. When you can hold your form together for a longer period of time, increased *speed* with a lower perceived exertion level becomes attainable. This is the by-product of combining efficient running form with a good distance base. But, if you bypass efficiency and distance for speed, you'll encounter injury and a setback in your entire running program.

There are about as many types of training programs as there are runners. All of them profess to be the best training program available to get you faster, or into great shape, or to the other end of a marathon. A training formula is like a recipe for cookies—if you follow the directions, you'll end up with cookies. But if ten people follow the same recipe, they'll end up with ten different batches of cookies. In the end, recipes are really only general guidelines.

Instead, I'm going to offer you some valuable guidelines for approaching a training program. You will be an active participant, assessing your current state and designing a program that suits your needs, not the ideals of other people.

Form, Distance, and Speed: The Three Developmental Stages of the ChiRunning Technique

The key principle is the Pyramid, shown by the illustration.

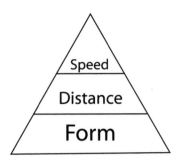

A solid foundation in good running technique will provide the necessary support for all that comes later. Your form is the base of the pyramid upon which increased distance, and then speed, will be supported. In short, your pyramid will be only as solid as the base upon which it is built. Remember the Pyramid? It's all about energy efficiency, which for ChiRunning is in the form.

FORM: OPENNESS TO CHANGE

As you begin to set up your ChiRunning program, bear in mind that most of the early emphasis should be directed toward form work. If you're a beginning runner, you'll start off by working mostly on your form and then slowly adding on distance. If you're a seasoned runner, it might be wise to give yourself a couple of months to hone in on your form and lighten up on specific pacing, distance, or race goals. Believe me, the sacrifice is well worth it.

Here's my favorite story about working on your form for long-term improvement. I will paraphrase an article that appeared in the August 14, 2000, issue of *Time* magazine. In 1997 Tiger Woods was at the top of the heap, winning the British Open, the U.S. Open, the PGA Championship, and the Masters, all at the ripe old age of 20. But after watching endless videos of himself, he came to the conclusion that although he was winning a lot of tournaments, his swing needed some pretty deep reworking. In his words, "My swing really sucks."

His coach told him that he could do it, but not to expect to win any golf tournaments for a while. In fact, the coach said that his swing would get worse before it got better. Tiger was willing to take that risk because he knew it was the only way he could realize long-term improvement.

As he spent the next nineteen months working on his swing, Tiger won only one tour event out of nineteen starts. Everybody was saying, "What happened to Tiger? He was so good." The press was writing him off as a flash in the pan, and fans became increasingly disappointed.

Then, one day in May 1999, when Tiger was preparing for the Byron Nelson Classic, he finally felt something happen in his swing. It was exactly what he'd been looking for, and the rest, as they say, is history. He then proceeded to win ten of the next fourteen events, going on to win the prestigious Grand Slam of golf at the age of 24.

He did it all by first taking a good long look at his form, setting himself the goal of improving his swing, and then meticulously doing everything in his power, physically and mentally, to improve his form. The two ChiRunning principles that stand out here are Gradual Progress (making small continuous improvements) and Nonidentification (not being afraid of what others will think).

If Tiger Woods was willing to make a form change, putting his whole career at risk, you might be willing to slow down your pace— maybe skip that upcoming race and get into working toward the long-term results that will keep you running well for a lifetime.

DISTANCE: INSTATING NEW HABITS

Many people have a particular distance in mind that they would like to accomplish. I respect that desire, because I have it, too. But as you might guess, the *distance* I'm talking about is concerned more with the means than the end. I like to talk about distance as a tool to deepen your knowledge of the focuses and your own body. Once again, the path becomes the goal.

A spiritual teacher once told me that if you want to establish new habits, you should repeat the desired habit every day for forty days, and it will become ingrained in your consciousness. In ChiRunning, distance is the means by which you institute new healthy habits in your running. It is by repeating and holding the form focuses over time and distance that they become ingrained in your running technique.

In ChiRunning, the goal is not to run farther; the goal is to run longer while maintaining good form. You might be able to run a 10K, but if you're in serious pain for half of it and don't even want to think about running another one for a long time, what is it worth? I'd rather see someone run 2 miles really well than beat herself up for 6.2. The true test of ChiRunning is in how long you can hold your running form together. It's about quality, not quantity.

Your mind and body work best as a team. Your mind, directing the show, introduces the new habit, while your body, through long-term constant repetition, learns to form a new "groove" in which to operate. After you begin to feel the correct motion, it will soon become a habit, and then it's *yours*. It is the workings of the mind that are being tested over long distances. If your mind is working well for you, your body will know what to do—to run efficiently over an extended distance.

The first step is to teach your mind to be as focused as possible, so it can direct your body. In practicing a new form focus, your mind will naturally go through periods of remembering the focus and then being distracted. When your mind becomes distracted—and it *will*—it'll stay distracted until you bring your focus back into play. This requires having some creative methods for waking yourself up out of your distraction. Here are a few reminders that I've used successfully.

- **Mile markers:** Every time you pass a mile marker or a significant landmark on your running course, let it be a reminder for you to refocus your mind.
- **A friend:** Run with a friend and tell her which focus(es) you are working on. Then ask her to remind you of your focus throughout your run.

- **Countdown timer:** This my favorite. I set it to beep every five minutes and direct my attention back to my focus whenever I hear that little beep.
- **Water stops:** Whenever you pause for a drink of water, whether you're in a race or out on your own, reinstate your focus when you start running again.

For example, you might head out the door with the intention of working on posture during your run. After doing a practice posture stance, you start running and focus on keeping your posture straight. After a mile, you remember that you were trying to keep your posture straight, and you haven't thought about it over the past few minutes. Not to worry. The nature of the mind is to drift, and your job is to train it to focus. Just bring your attention back to the focus, make the necessary physical adjustments, and continue on with your run. Each time you return to your focus, renew your intention to hold it. Repetitive reminders from your mind will train your body to hold a focus longer. This is not any different from how a meditation instructor would teach you to meditate. If you're sitting and observing your breath, *that's* your focus; whenever you find your mind wandering, you drop what you're thinking about and return to your breath. ChiRunning focus is like doing a running meditation. As you learn to hold each ChiRunning focus for a longer distance, you'll be able to add in a second focus, and then a third, until eventually you can run with many happening simultaneously.

It's like learning a language. You begin by learning the vocabulary words (the focuses). Then you learn how to put the words together into sentences (doing a workout). When you become adept at making sentences, you can write a composition (the equivalent of running a race, an organized event, or a long run). Finally, when you've mastered the use of vocabulary and syntax, you can try your hand at writing poetry. In running terms, this means that no matter what comes up on your run, you can respond with the right mix of focuses and movements— turning your running into an art form. Why do you think T'ai Chi is called a martial art? It's because a T'ai Chi master can respond to any situation in a way that is instantaneous, creative, and correct. That's poetry.

SPEED: THE ICING ON THE CAKE

As much as I downplay the need for speed, running all out is one of my favorite things to do. It's exhilarating and fun. When you have your form together and your body is comfortable with running, all of the training comes together and speed happens. Here are four letters from clients who express their delight with running fast and its apparent ease. The first letter is from a triathlete who came to me because he dreaded running and wanted to develop a better relationship with it.

Danny,

I wanted to tell you about a "breakthrough" run I had on Friday. As you know it was an absolutely gorgeous day, so I decided to go for an "aggressive" run up Mount Tam (2,500-foot elevation gain in 6 miles). I originally thought that I would run a 1:30 out-and-back up Shaver Grade, but two things changed my plans dramatically. First was the wonderful frame of mind that the sunshine put me in, which served to provide me boundless energy. Second was a feeling of weightlessness, which came about as I constantly reinforced the techniques I had learned in my lessons with you. I felt as if I were just "renting" the ground for brief moments instead of pushing off of it. I ended up running (at a decent clip) all the way up Eldridge Grade to East Peak. After a 10-minute break at the top, I began to worry about how I would hold up on the descent, since I was a bit fatigued. As I started down from the parking lot and onto Eldridge Grade, I began thinking again about the things you taught me (keep the calves silent, arm swing, weight forward), and suddenly I was simply gliding over the treacherous rocks at the top of Eldridge, and my run took on a Zenlike feel. By the time I got down to the Indian Fire Road intersection, I was in a near sprint, which continued until I exited at the Natalie Coffin Greene gate. I finished feeling stronger and more in control than when I started $2^{1}/_{2}$ hours earlier.

This season I am placing a much greater emphasis on my running, since it has always been my weak point. I have run more in the last six months than ever before, so I was probably due for some kind of breakthrough run. However, this one was in no small part a result of really feeling all of the ChiRunning elements come together to achieve running nirvana. While I won't go so far as to say that I now love the portion of the triathlon that I once dreaded, a couple more runs like this one, and who knows?

Thanks for making possible this highlight in my athletic (as well as personal) life. Regards, *Evan*

This next letter is from a person who wrote to me after only one hour-long session of coaching.

Dear Danny,

My name is Chris, and I had the pleasure of your company and instruction last Thursday morning. The introduction to ChiRunning was nothing less than life-changing. It makes so much sense, and for someone who loves to run as much as I do, it affords me the real vision of being able to run for the rest of my life, injury-free.

Not only does ChiRunning excite me with its potential to avoid injuries, but since our time together, I've been playing with it and been amazed at the results. While I'm sure I'm not doing it very well, what I have been doing has netted wonderful benefits. When I normally complete a run, my calves and quads are tight, and I can really feel them as I stretch. Now I barely notice the muscles and any soreness. There is even an energizing afterward.

What really surprised me was the improvement in my time and distance. While this is all new and takes focus [and] concentration . . . the effort I used to put out is now redirected, and instead of running "up and down," I'm simply leaning. The outcome of that is a stark and marked improvement of my normal pace. What used to be a relaxed 8-minute-pace daily run has turned into a 6:50-to-7-minute pace. I've been fitting in another mile on each of my daily runs in the same amount of time I used to run. I decided to see how ChiRunning held up on a longer run, so I tried it on my 12-mile run this weekend. Well, I ran it in 1:24 minutes . . . a 12-minute improvement over the week before! Mind-blowing!! Today I played with it at the track and paced myself at 6:50/mile pace without much more of an effort than I used to put out running the old way.

    Take care, Danny, and thanks for your time. *Chris*

This letter is from a woman who took a full-day ChiRunning form clinic and expressed concern about running a half-marathon the following day. I told her not to worry, to listen to her body and have a good time. She is a recreational runner, a mother, and a day-care worker. Here's her report of the results.

Hi, Danny,

I attended your workshop last Saturday at UCLA. I did the half-marathon on Sunday and did GREAT! I did something strange to both my calves on Saturday, so they were both very sore going into the event. I started out really slow, kept talking to my body, practiced some of the technique, and enjoyed the moment. Well, guess what? I broke my best time by 13 minutes [a drop of 1 minute per mile in pace]. I ran more than I expected, and before I knew it, my legs were warmed up and not in pain.

    Sincerely, *Cheri*

The next letter is an example of how enjoyable speed can be when you're not thinking about it. This man previously had severe leg pains whenever he ran over a half hour.

Hello Danny,

I'm writing this e-mail to share some good news. About two weeks ago, I ran the inaugural US Half Marathon in the city. Things that helped me out during the run: creating as light a foot strike as I can, the correct elbow swing, and the all-important lean. And now the icing on the cake. I bettered my timing by 26 minutes, from 2:39 to 2:13 [a previous pace of 12:08 minutes per mile versus a new pace of 10:09]. Thank you so much. You helped me realize that running can be fun and pain-free. It's a long road to perfection. I have "miles" to go, but at least I'm having a lot of fun doing it.

    Thank you so much! *Anil*

Speed comes last in the progression of *Form, Distance, and Speed* because it is totally dependent on the quality of its two predecessors, form and distance. Speed is the by-product of your ability to do the necessary focuses in the right proportion. In the end, your technique will support your speed. This is the Pyramid in action—the end result (more speed) is supported by the foundation (your technique).

In ChiRunning, speed doesn't come from pushing, it comes from an increased ability to focus and relax; it should not be the solitary goal of any workout. Running faster can be fun, especially when it is the by-product of a well-done process.

CREATING A RUNNING PROGRAM

Going on vacation, for me, is a sacred event. It doesn't happen that often, so it's crucial that I spend much of the scarcely allotted time enjoying myself. Vacations are the best metaphor I can think of to introduce the concept of planning ahead, because most people have some experience with them, and the subject usually brings up lots of emotions, because really enjoyable and enriching vacations rarely happen.

How would you plan your vacation so there would be a minimum of glitches? You might want to think back to some of your more memorable hassles and plan to avoid repeating the same experiences—like the time you booked a week in the tropics at a bargain price, only to realize when you got there that it was their monsoon season . . . or the time you weren't aware there would be a Hell's Angels convention at your campground during the week of your stay. Maybe you've learned that having a full day at home before going back to work has made all the difference.

How do you get ready for a vacation? What steps do you follow year after year that have worked for you? What have you learned from past vacation failures that you wouldn't repeat? What are your larger goals or objectives? The design process should be no less for your running program, especially since you'll probably spend more days each year running than vacationing.

This section is devoted to helping you design a running program that really works for you—on all levels. Building a good program should take into account:

(1) Your present condition
(2) Your aspirations
(3) The rest of your life
(4) The specifics of each run

By following these four steps you will be able to develop a well-planned, well-rounded program that will be organized, sequential, and in tune with your body's needs and capabilities.

Set yourself up with a running journal and take notes on your answers. A journal can serve multiple functions, as mentioned in Chapter 5:

- You'll have a record of where you started from. It's important and motivating to look back to your beginnings and acknowledge the changes that have taken place.
- You'll learn over time what works and what doesn't work, and what you need to focus on if you have a repeating issue.
- You can keep a list of your intentions, past and present, so you can remind yourself what you are currently working on and why you chose those focuses. This will keep you on track with the process of improving your running form.
- The process of writing gets you in touch with and affirms what you really want.

Assess Your Current State

It is important to begin with an honest personal assessment of where you're beginning, so there are no illusions about what you can and can't do relative to your running. In other words, start from where you're at, not from somewhere else. Nobody likes to encounter the old one-step-forward-three-steps-back scenario. Therefore, spend time assessing your current physical condition and mental attitude up front so restarts or setbacks are kept to a minimum. You can come up with a great running program, but if your present state isn't taken into account, it could end up being too ambitious, too time-consuming, or beyond your current capabilities in some way.

There are three parts to the assessment process: physical, mental, and your ability with the ChiRunning skills.

THE PHYSICAL ASSESSMENT

Here are some questions to ask yourself as you sit down to design your program. These questions are guidelines. Your physical assessment will be specific to your physical state. Remember, this is for your eyes only, so be as honest as you can.

- What is your current physical state? (Are you overweight, asthmatic, under any doctor's care concerning physical activity, do you have high blood pressure?)
- Do you have any aches or pains?
- Do you have any injuries?
- How many minutes do you run each week? (Not miles— remember, we're also working on Nonidentification here.)
- How many minutes is your current longest run?

THE MENTAL ASSESSMENT: THINKING/FEELING

Ponder some of the following questions and see what pops up in your head. Getting a clear sense of your thoughts and feelings regarding your program will allow you to tailor a running program to fit your specific needs.

- How much a part of your life do you want running to occupy?
- Why do you really run?
- What do you want from running?
- Do you feel better training with a group? Alone? With a partner?
- How good are you at being self-motivated, with staying on a training program?

- Would you like to achieve a certain distance or pace?
- Is there a specific race you'd like to train for?
- What are your fears around running?

ASSESS YOUR CHIRUNNING SKILLS

Once you've read Chapter 4 and started to practice the ChiRunning technique, do four or five runs and then evaluate your strengths and weaknesses with doing the ChiRunning technique. Leaning might come naturally to you, but relaxing might not. This is best done immediately after each run, and should be a regular practice. Get out your running journal and write down any visualizations or reminders that worked particularly well, along with areas where you experienced some level of difficulty. In this way you'll be consistently assessing your current ChiRunning skills and working on new ones. I always have at least one area of focus that I pay attention to during any given run.

While writing this book, I went through a three-week time period during which my lower back got stiff from sitting and writing at the computer for hours on end. So every time I went out for a run, I'd focus on relaxing my pelvis and sacrum the entire time. Downhill running accentuates the rotation of the pelvis and sacrum, so I'd head out looking for the longest gradual hill I could find. I'd take my time climbing up the hill, and on the way back down, I would let my stride open up and my hips relax. After a couple of miles of downhill running, I'd return home relaxed and ready for another stint at the computer . . . problem solved.

Later in this chapter I will describe various types of workouts and list the specific focuses that best match the workout. If you find yourself slow to pick up one of the focuses, I suggest doing a run that accentuates it. The body learns best through repetition, which shortens the time it takes to learn the focus.

Questions to Ask Yourself

Which form focuses are the hardest for me to do?

What are the weak areas of my ChiRunning technique?

Do I clearly understand the instructions for each focus?

The answers to these questions will provide you with a clearer view of what to work on during your run.

SET BODY-ORIENTED GOALS

Now that you have assessed your current state, you can readily determine some legitimate goals that will truly serve your best interests. By "legitimate" I mean goals that have a depth of thinking and feeling behind them—and ones that won't throw off the balance of your life to accomplish.

There is definitely something to be said for setting goals, but be careful that they don't slip into being result-oriented. That internal conversation might sound something like "I want to run faster than my neighbor." Or "I want to win that race." Whereas a body-oriented goal would be one that wells up from inside. The goal should also be within your capacity to manifest in a healthy way, given the right conditions and a realistic time frame. There's nothing wrong with a goal if you're listening to your body and asking it a reasonable request.

Your goals must come from your body and from your present reality, not from other peoples' idea of what's cool. Don't think outside of yourself. Let your goals be an expression of who you are, not something that will impress someone or earn praise. Do something because you deeply want to, not because you're driven to. Here are some synonyms for "driven" that I've come across in various word searches: to be made, to be necessitated, to be obliged, to be ordered or required, to have to, and, everybody's favorite, should. All of these synonyms leave one with the sense of being *externally* motivated. A result-oriented goal might sound like "I want to run a 6-minute mile." Translated into a body-oriented goal, it would sound more like "I want to be a faster runner." The former statement holds me to a specific path that will be considered successful only if I run a 6-minute mile. If a 6:23 mile is the fastest I'll ever run, I'll never be totally happy, because I never reached my goal.

On the other hand, the goal of being a faster runner automatically puts the emphasis on the *process*, because being fast is a relative statement. Faster than what? Faster than who? Faster than I am now? Stating that I want to be faster directs my attention to what my *body* will have to go through to achieve that goal. This is how the emphasis is taken off the goal and put onto the process.

I definitely have goals, but they're all body-oriented. Here are a few of the ones I've worked on with success over the years:

- To run with no knee pain
- To finish well in ultramarathons, training no more than 35 miles per week
- To run without injury
- To finish my runs feeling good

The *process* is the most valuable goal, and these are all process-oriented goals. It's great to have the goal of running a 5K, a 10K, or a marathon, but be sure to allow yourself enough training time to really enjoy the process and get something of value from it.

Think of any goals that you'd like to achieve and write them down in your running journal. If you sense that there are any result-oriented goals popping up in the list, just move them to a separate list ... for later disposal. Here are some more suggestions for body-oriented goals: ease of movement, fluidity, no injuries, injury recovery, increased fitness level, improved diet, feeling good about yourself, getting outdoors.

When you have goals that come from your deepest self, they're a great opportunity to practice the principle of Cotton and Steel. As you work to come from your center (steel), you learn not to be ruled by what others might think (cotton: that which is outside of you). It's good to be informed by others, but final decisions and actions are best when they come from within.

SCHEDULING YOUR PROGRAM

Now that you've done your homework of assessment and goal setting, it's time to put it all together into a workable schedule. You'll need to get out your running journal and your calendar. The basic idea is to come up with a workout schedule that won't throw the rest of your life out of balance. I mean, who needs a life that's more difficult? If you're starting a new running program, or adding running to an established fitness program, these questions will guide you through the process of carving out the time. If you already have a running program, the questions will help you refine it.

In your running journal write down your answers to the following questions.

(1) How many days a week do you want to run? (I recommend at least 3 but no more than 6 days a week, if running is your main form of exercise. It's easier to keep a momentum going with your workouts if they're not too spread out and if you're not running all the time.)

(2) Given that number of days, which specific days of the week work best to support it?

(3) On each of those chosen days, how many minutes could you dedicate to a workout? Be sure to include any travel time and transition times, along with your actual running time. Don't crunch your time if you can help it.

(4) On each of those chosen days, what time would you be most likely to guarantee a workout would happen?

(5) Go immediately to your calendar and block out these times.

These questions require you to take into account what is happening in the rest of your life, especially around the time when your run is scheduled to happen. Step 5 requires that you hold yourself responsible to do what you say you're going to do. These steps are the backbone of a consistent running program. The whole idea is to develop a successful plan that blends seamlessly with the rest of your life.

Treat your workouts as appointments. If someone calls you, asking to get together during one of these blocks of time, just say that you have something scheduled and ask if there's another time you could meet. By giving your running program the priority that it deserves, you'll be practicing the principle of Cotton and Steel—gathering to your center and letting go of peripheral things.

THE TRAINING PALETTE

Now that you know how many times a week you'll be running, here's where you'll determine which types of runs to plug into your schedule. There are five types of runs that will cover the whole spectrum of training situations. Even though you will be practicing many of the ChiRunning focuses on each run, certain focuses are particularly suited to certain runs. Each run will have a unique set of characteristics that contribute to the whole of your technique. When the ChiRunning focuses become an integral part of your running, you will have a built-in set of tools to use in any situation.

THE WELL-ROUNDED RUNNING PROGRAM

A well-rounded running program is one that will condition your body, build core strength, improve your circulation, increase your range of motion, increase your aerobic capacity, strengthen your heart, help to relieve stress, and generally improve your physical, mental, and spiritual well-being. The chart on the next page shows three sample running programs. Level I is for beginners and those coming back from injury who want to build a solid base in their conditioning and running technique. Level II is for intermediate runners who are looking to improve their conditioning base and reduce their PEL. Level III is for seasoned runners and competitors wanting to improve their conditioning base, maximize their efficiency, and increase their speed.

Full descriptions of each of the listed runs immediately follow the chart.

INTERVALS: SPEED AND FORM

I recommend two types of intervals—speed intervals and form intervals.

Form Intervals

I highly recommend this workout for beginning runners or for those coming back after a long break. This is a fun workout. In fact, you can always substitute this run for a scheduled fun run. For the

Sample Running Programs

Day	Level I	Level II	Level III
1	Off	Speed intervals or form intervals	Speed intervals
2	Fun run or form intervals	Hill run	Hill run
3	Off	Off	Tempo run
4	Fun run or form intervals	Tempo run	Off
5	Off	Off	Fun run or form intervals
6	Fun run or form intervals	Long run	Long run
7	Off or fun run	Off	Off

duration of your run, you will alternate between focusing and not focusing—one minute on, one minute off, one minute on, one minute off, until you finish. Before your run, go over your list of focuses that you feel a need to work on.

- If you have a sports watch with a repeat countdown timer, set it to beep every minute. Focus on one aspect of your technique for a minute, then relax and don't focus for a minute.
- Once you're warmed up and running at a comfortable pace, start your countdown timer. When the beep goes off, bring all of your attention to the focus that you picked and do everything in your power to hold it for the entire minute *without a single lapse in concentration*. It's only a minute, so try hard to stay with it. When you hear the next beep, drop the focus, relax, and enjoy yourself for a minute.
- When the beep goes off again, go back to concentrating on your specific focus for the next minute.

- Repeat this pattern of alternating focus with relaxation for the rest of your run.
- If you've picked two focuses, do one of them for the first third of your run, and do the second one for the second third. In the final third, try to hold both focuses at the same time for one-minute intervals.

For beginners, this is one of the most efficient ways to learn the individual focuses, because in a thirty-minute run, you'll practice engaging a specific focus fifteen times!

The three focuses that I recommend starting with are:

(1) Holding your posture straight
(2) Leaning from your feet
(3) Picking up your feet as you run

Speed Intervals

This workout is a favorite because it's the most fun. It's an exercise in instant gratification, because I'm not *trying* to run faster. I'm trying to hold all of my form focuses together, then using my times as a confirmation. Speed is *not* the primary goal of this workout. There are so many other things that are more important to work on that thinking of speed would only serve as a distraction. The simple definition of "interval" is a period of highly focused running followed by a period of nonfocused running at a restful pace.

Speed is a by-product of proper form. Here is another type of form interval in which you set up the right conditions for speed to happen. No matter what level of runner you are, speed intervals should be undertaken only when you feel comfortable with holding the focuses. Here are the key focuses to work on during your intervals.

- Start off slowly, and *very* gradually increase your lean throughout the length of the interval.
- Relax your lower body (hips, pelvis, and legs) as you lean more.
- Allow your stride to lengthen behind you as you increase your lean.

- Maintain a steady cadence at all times (85 to 90 strides per minute each leg).
- Engage your upper body more at higher speeds. Keep your shoulders relaxed and your elbows swinging fully out the back.
- Relax your lower back as you run faster. Let your abdominals hold your lean in place.
- Use your core muscles more and your legs less.
- Pick up your feet higher, but keep your knees low as you increase your lean. Don't pick up your knees, or you'll be using unnecessary effort.

It is a prime opportunity to practice the principle of Gradual Progress because you're always working from slow to fast, from small to big,

Let's say, for example, that you would like to increase your basic running speed. Pick one day each week to go to your local track and do some 400-meter intervals (400 meters is one lap around most tracks). This means that you will focus on one or more of the above focuses for a lap, then rest for a lap. Repeat this sequence 4 to 10 times, depending on your level of conditioning. If you don't know how many intervals you should do, let your body tell you. Start off with four and then Body Sense whether or not you can handle more. Listen carefully to your body, and you'll know when you're done.

Follow the Gradual Progress rule and run your first interval the slowest. It's tempting to take off fast on the first one, since you usually feel fresh at the beginning of a workout. Don't be tempted. People often start off with a fast first interval, then get a little slower with each successive one until the last one, in which they barely hang on to any semblance of form. Additionally, they start each interval as fast as they can, burning out most of their energy during the first half of the lap and struggling to keep the same speed at the finish. It doesn't matter what speed your first interval is as long as it feels comfortable. So be sure to start slow enough not to exhaust all your energy at the outset.

You'll get a much better workout by letting each interval be a loosening exercise for the next one. As your workout progresses, every additional interval will be a little faster, not because you're pushing harder but because your joints and ligaments are looser and more relaxed.

Beginning slowly allows you to work on your form focuses and think about what you're doing, to sense what's right and not right. Each interval becomes a stepping-stone for the next one to be even better. Take what you've learned from each interval and apply it to the next one, and you'll constantly improve throughout the workout.

When you've done your last interval, jog a couple of easy laps and congratulate yourself on a job well done.

LSD RUN

I look forward to doing the long slow distance run each week—it's like looking forward to hanging out with an old friend. It's pure enjoyment! If my week has been particularly stressful, I can head into the woods knowing that I'll be a different person when I arrive back at my car. It's that predictable. It's a time for me, a time to let the dust settle and gather my thoughts. I resolve world problems, watch the seasons change, or just explore new territory. My mind is a clean slate when I take off. I'm not concerned about speed or distance; it's just time on my feet that I'm looking for.

The long run is a perfect opportunity to spend lots of time working on your focuses. I would say that relaxing is the most important thing to focus on. Do a Body Scan (see Chapter 7) every 10 minutes, and watch for any place in your body that feels tense or tight. Then focus on relaxing that particular area. If you hold the focus of relaxing for the entire run, you will finish your runs feeling like you just got a great massage. This level of relaxation can be brought into all of your runs. Other focuses to practice on your long run are cadence, gears, and posture, but not speed.

This run does wonders for building your aerobic capacity by triggering your body to produce more extensive capillary beds. That's how oxygen gets into your muscles from your bloodstream. As your muscles improve oxygen uptake, all your runs will go better, because more of the oxygen from your lungs gets to your muscles, creating better efficiency. For those of you who want to be faster, the long run is what gives you the aerobic base to apply to speed training later on.

How long should a long run be? As long as you want, given the current capacity of your body and whatever amount of time you can afford. How much time would you like? If you're a beginning runner, your long run might be 30 minutes. When I was training to run the Leadville Trail 100 Mile Endurance Run, my long run was 40 miles every Sunday. That earned me permanent status in the lunatic-fringe category of runners. Now, 3 hours once a week, year round, feels just fine. Your long run should not be so long as to leave you wiped out. You should end your run feeling pleasantly tired.

FUN RUN

A fun run is just what it sounds like. When you've had a tough day or a sleepless night, or when you notice that you've been taking yourself way too seriously lately, it's time to go for a fun run. It can also be used as a recovery run following a long run or a fast run.

Go explore a new area.

Go window-shopping.

Go to a beautiful nature spot.

Take a friend on a tour of your favorite running route.

Leave your watch at home, and don't think about pace or distance. The emphasis of the run is on letting yourself relax mentally. Don't take anything seriously (especially yourself); just have fun.

HILL RUN

A hill run can be of any intensity, from mellow, rolling country roads to steep trails. Use your best judgment. If you've never run hills and would like to, find easy ones to start with and run up only as far as is comfortable, then turn around and come back down. Like speed workouts, hills shouldn't be done until you get familiar and comfortable with holding the basic ChiRunning form focuses. If you run on hills when you're learning to do ChiRunning, your body will default to the way you used to run, thus complicating and lengthening the learning process. Since running up and down hills is a skill unto itself, I have given a full explanation of hill-running techniques in Chapter 7, under "Special Circumstances" (see page 175).

TEMPO RUN

A tempo run is the only run in this series of workouts that builds in both distance and speed. Seasoned runners use it for race practice. The distance is generally 4 to 8 miles, depending on your conditioning level. I don't recommend this workout for beginning runners or for anyone who doesn't have a good working knowledge of the ChiRunning focuses.

The object is to start off at a comfortable pace and slowly increase your lean over the length of the run. It might feel a bit faster than you're used to, because you're trying to do negative splits: Each mile gets progressively faster, so your mile split times get smaller . . . hence, negative splits. If you're training for a race and you want to average an 8:52 pace, you would start off running slower than your average pace and end the run going faster than your average pace (as shown below).

Mile 1: 9:00
Mile 2: 8:55
Mile 3: 8:50
Mile 4: 8:45

Your average pace for the 4 miles would be 8:52. You can adjust the numbers to fit your own training needs. The most difficult part of the workout is doing the math.

A tempo run is a lesson in technique, not strength. The goal is to feel the *same* perceived effort level and the *same* cadence throughout even though your speed increases with each mile.

"You're nuts! How can that be possible?" you might say.

Well, I won't argue with you about whether or not I'm nuts. But it is entirely possible to do this workout as I've proposed. It's a matter of using your lean while relaxing your body, and that's it in a nutshell.

Here's how the concept works. In ChiRunning, the more you lean your body forward, the more important it is to hold your posture straight so you don't bend at the waist. This will allow your feet to land just behind your center of gravity. As you lean more, your stride will open up behind you, not in front of you. The best way to lengthen your stride is to relax from the waist down. This will allow your spine to gain a slight twist as you counterrotate your body, which in turn allows your legs to swing more freely from your hips. When you relax your lower legs, your ankles, calves, and shins aren't working, either. There's not much happening below the waist except relaxation of all your body parts.

To keep your cadence uniform, use a small electronic metronome. This isn't just a recommendation, it's a requirement if you really want to learn to lengthen your stride. I set mine for 90 beats per minute and start it up as soon as I take my first step into my run. If you're used to running with a slower cadence, set the metronome for a minimum of 85 beats per minute. The best place to do this run is on a track. That way you can pace yourself by checking your timer every lap.

If you've never done a run like this and you don't know what pace you should run, let your body tell you. Jog a couple of warm-up laps at a very easy pace, do your Body Looseners, and then start your run at a pace that is slightly easier than your normal cruising speed. If you have a stopwatch that records split times, hit the split button after each lap. The next lap should be 1 second faster. That's not a lot. Subsequently each lap will be a second faster until you've done the last lap. After 4 miles you will have run 16 laps, so your last lap should be 16 seconds faster than the first.

This is a *very* slow rate of increase in speed, so watch the timer closely. If you run the first lap in 2:00 minutes and the second lap in 1:55, you can let off on the gas pedal a little in the next lap. This is one of the best Body Sensing exercises, because you have to listen very closely to your body and make tiny adjustments in speed. Nothing drastic here. It's one of my favorite runs, because I like the challenge of seeing how close I can come to the target time for each lap. If I come across the lap marker at 1:45, I know on the next lap I'll be looking for 1:44 to show up on the watch. It's fun, in a different kind of way, and very challenging.

To change your speed, you will be using your lean as a gas pedal. If you need to go faster, you'll lean slightly more. If you need to slow down, come back upright a bit. If you do a run like this once a week, you'll be a master at pacing in no time, which will be a huge advantage in races. Everyone in your pace group will shoot away from the start line, and you'll be a little ways back in the pack, smiling, knowing that you will pass them all later.

Since each of the five types of runs offers its own benefits to your overall ChiRunning technique, here is a table showing which form focuses are best learned in each of the five workouts.

The Five Workouts and Their Relative Focuses

Type of Run	1 Tempo	2 Hill	3 Interval	4 Long	5 Fun Run or Recovery
Type of Focus	Run	Run	Run	Run	Run
Posture	X	X		X	X
Lean	X		X	X	
Cadence	X	X		X	X
Gears	X	X	X		
Arm swing	X	X	X		
Hip swing	X	X		X	X
Core strength	X	X	X		
Aerobic capacity				X	X
Cardiovascular		X	X		

WHAT ABOUT CROSS-TRAINING?

People often ask me if they should do any cross-training for their running. My response is, if you think you need to build muscles, it's best to build them in the motion they'll be used while running. I believe in core-muscle training, but I don't believe in weight training for running. Building muscles that you don't use while running will only increase your muscle mass, creating more weight you'll have to carry around. No thanks, I'll pass on that. I practice T'ai Chi for cross-training my core muscles and focusing my mind.

Do your training on the run. If you want to build muscle, run more, but don't spend your time on weights unless you need strength for something else. If your doctor tells you it's necessary to build stronger muscles so you can recover from an injury, fine. But be sure you're also working to improve your running form, since it's what probably caused the injury to begin with. Here's an example of what I mean.

Let's say your feet turn out when you run, creating knee problems. Your physical therapist tells you to strengthen your adductor muscles so your feet point forward more when you run. Now, you can either go to the gym and do tons of adductor-strengthening exercises, or you can do the following.

Go out running, and swing your knee straight forward with every step, not flaring it out to the side as you normally would. Run like you're on a tightrope, and make your knees swing close to your centerline by holding in on your adductor muscles. If your cadence is 85 to 90 strides per minute, and you're running at a 10 minute-mile pace, you'll be flexing those adductors over 2,500 times in 30 minutes of running, without having set foot inside of a gym.

If your ligaments and tendons aren't very flexible, or if certain muscles needed in your running are weak, enhance your workouts with specific cross-training until your body can get up to speed. But the most effective way for your whole body to work well is to strengthen and stretch it *while you're running.*

PROGRAM UPGRADES: WHEN, HOW, HOW MUCH

For anything to evolve to its next appropriate level of existence, for it to grow, it needs to be prodded or stretched out of its state of equilibrium into a state of imbalance, at which time the forces of Nature are engaged to create a new state of equilibrium at a new level.

If this premise is true, then balance and growth cannot exist simultaneously, because balance implies a state of equilibrium, or non-movement, and growth implies a state of movement. This may all sound very heady and esoteric, but it applies directly to your running. Here's how.

Let's say you've been religiously doing all of your ChiRunning focuses, and you've gotten to the point where you can run at a nice relaxed pace, whistling pop tunes. Your body has been so used to running at this pace for so long that your runs feel pretty relaxed and effortless. In essence, you've reached a nice state of equilibrium. You might feel at home and balanced in this state. So you say to yourself, "This is okay, but I'd like to get a little faster." What do you do?

As explained in Chapter 4, if you want to go faster, all you have to do is *lean* more. So then you go out for your next run and try to lean more. What happens? If you're doing it right, you'll feel like you're tipping more forward than you're used to. You're off balance a bit and it'll probably feel somewhat uncomfortable. But with each progressive run it gets easier because Nature is doing its part by providing you with stronger abdominal muscles to handle this new angle of lean. After some weeks or maybe months, you find yourself running along with a new lean, still whistling pop tunes, just like you used to except now you're running faster! In essence, your running evolves because you introduce a state of imbalance where one hadn't existed before. Your body makes the necessary adjustments, and presto, you end up in a new state of balance that is a step above your original state—you've grown!

That's what growth is all about. It doesn't come when things are status quo. It happens only when something new is introduced, forcing every integral part to adjust. This is a universal law that can be applied on any level of life, whether it's expanding a business or helping a shy person become a better public speaker.

In the case of expanding a business, somebody either has to work more hours or sell more product or better organize himself. You name it. Something beyond the normal state of existence has to happen for something progressive to come about. Then things will begin to fall into place that support the new condition until it becomes balanced again, but in an expanded version.

A shy person will remain a shy person unless he or she initiates a state of imbalance. That might require putting oneself into social circumstances where one is challenged to mingle and talk more than normal. When a shy person has to engage more, it might feel awkward (a state of imbalance). But if that person does it regularly and often, it will get easier and easier until the former state of imbalance goes away and a new state of balance is achieved—one in which that same person may feel comfortable in a crowd. That growth never would have happened if that person hadn't dived into the crowd to begin with.

I don't want to imply just because you're in a state of imbalance that you're growing, but the possibility of growth is there. Too many people live most of their lives in an *un*balanced state and never get anywhere.

To get this law to work for you, you must come from a balanced state and make a conscious choice to improve it. *You* choose when to stretch yourself and create the necessary state of imbalance (think Tiger Woods). Your job is to make the adjustments required to move you forward (such as really working on holding that lean). Once you choose to grow, you'll be amazed at how the forces of Nature line up to help you complete the job. Balance and growth are two of the main principles that keep Nature ticking along in that wonderful way.

THE PHILOSOPHY OF UPGRADES: AN ADVANCED LESSON IN THE PRINCIPLE OF BALANCE

One of the most important ways to build your running program safely is to know when and how much to upgrade. As your conditioning increases, your breath rate will relax, and your core muscles won't be as tired. Maintaining a consistent lean won't be as difficult. Your shoulders and hips will feel looser and your footsteps lighter. As all of these improvements take place, your running will feel easier, and at some point you will have a choice to make. You can either plateau for a period of time, or you can upgrade your program.

A *plateau* is an important and natural part of any growth process. It is the period of time necessary for your physical development to catch up with the changes taking place in your running form. You body needs time to get used to the fact that some muscles are being used more and some less. It's an adjustment on the cellular level, and it takes time. My 3-year-old daughter goes through growth spurts in which she'll gain an inch in a month, and then there'll be no change for a couple of weeks while the rest of her body catches up with her bone growth.

An *upgrade* is any increase in your current running program beyond what you are currently doing. Upgrading your program is a bigger deal than you might think. Any quantitative increase in your speed, distance, technique, or number of runs will increase duress to your body—namely, your muscles, ligaments, tendons, bones, heart, and lungs. For this reason it is crucial that you hold your upgrades to no more than two per week.

General Guidelines for Upgrading a Running Program

- Don't make more than two upgrades of any kind per week.
- Don't add more than 15 to 30 seconds on to an interval.
- Don't add more than 15 minutes (or 10% additional mileage) to a long run each week.
- If you increase the number of intervals, run the earlier ones slightly slower.
- If you increase the speed at which you run your intervals, decrease the total number, then slowly build the number weekly while maintaining your new speed.
- If you happen to have a good run when you unexpectedly run faster or farther than usual, don't follow it with any scheduled upgrades. Postpone them until the following week.

Upgrades that are not well thought out and prepared for are the number one cause of running injuries. This is called overtraining, the general term used to describe a level of running, beyond which your body is capable. It occurs in all classes of runners, from beginners to elites. If you try to run 2 miles on your very first run, you could be easily injured in a number of ways. If there are weaknesses in your running form, the potential for injury magnifies as the miles increase. Build slowly and let your body knowledge grow gradually until you can add upgrades without defaulting back into how you used to run.

If you're a beginning runner, your first upgrades will be in more minutes to your runs. The next upgrade will be form intervals (see page 138).

As you get a clearer understanding and body experience of the ChiRunning focuses, you will be able to sense within yourself what you most need to upgrade. Go by feel.

Here are some examples of upgrades and what each would entail.

- **Increase the speed of a specific run.** This is done by increasing your lean angle (increased abdominal work). Look at it as an adjustment in your core muscle usage, not in your leg usage. This upgrade not only increases your speed, but your stride gets longer, too. To accommodate a longer stride, you'll have to relax your hips, pelvis, and lower back. It's the domino effect. If you change anything "upstream" at your core, be prepared to adjust everything "downstream" that is affected.
- **Increase the number of interval repeats.** Increase your interval workout by no more than one interval per week, and add one only if your body says it's okay. (See "How to Tell When You Need an Upgrade," page 152.)
- **Increase the amount of time of each interval.** This will be between 15 and 30 seconds, depending on the length of your intervals. If you're doing one-minute intervals, increase only 15 seconds per interval. If you're doing 2-minute intervals, you can add on 30 seconds.
- **Increase the time of a run.** This generally translates into additional mileage. If it's a long run, check on your body a mile before your projected finish time and see how you feel. If you're feeling reasonably fresh, you can add 10 to 15 minutes to your run. If you're feeling a little tired, you're done for the day. Just stop at the predetermined time.
- **Increase the steepness or length of a hill run.** Your hill runs should be at a comfortable pace. They're among the trickiest workouts to tell how to upgrade, because they involve a mix of distance and elevation gain/loss. If you plan to go out for what you know to be a longer hill run than you're used to, take it very easy in the

early miles, on both the uphills *and* on the downhills. It's easy to overexert yourself on a hilly run, so pace yourself and save your best energy for the later miles.

- **Increase the number of your weekly runs.** This is a big step and not to be taken lightly. Any additional weekly run should always be a fun run at first—nothing challenging—you want to test the waters. Be aware that it's not just your running program that will be affected but the rest of your life. Allow yourself a couple of weeks to transition into the additional day per week before introducing any specific theme into the run (i.e., speed, distance, hills, etc.).

- **Change the nature of your runs.** Any new theme that you bring into one of your runs (i.e., changing from three five-mile flat runs per week to one hill run, one fun run, and one long run) deserves a nice slow introduction. Balance and Gradual Progress are the best principles to follow here.

How to Tell When You Need an Upgrade

Body Sensing, Body Sensing, Body Sensing. You guessed it—you can do it when your body says it's okay. If you try to push an upgrade before your body is ready, you're asking for trouble. Any upgrades need to be proposed by your mind but ratified by your body, kind of like the House and Senate.

The best time to check in with your body is toward the end of the run that you plan to upgrade. As you approach the close of your scheduled workout, ask yourself, "Could I do another ___ right now?" (Fill in the blank with the appropriate increment: 1 interval, 1 mile, 15 minutes, 30 seconds, whatever.) If you listen carefully to your body, it will give you one of three responses when you ask it to do more:

(A) "Sure, no problem."
(B) "Yeah, I *could* do it. I'm a little tired, but I think I've got it in me."
(C) "No way. I'm outta here!"

If your body answers with A or B, you have the green light for an upgrade. Anything in the C range is out of the question. Give it another week before asking again.

Even if you have a scheduled upgrade in a given week, you should upgrade only if it's appropriate to your conditioning.

The beauty of this method is that it has the built-in safety mechanism of Body Sensing, which, if used properly, will never allow you to be injured due to a premature upgrade. Warning: Body Sensing is easily cut off by the ego. Keep a good back-and-forth dialogue happening with your body, and it will always let you know what's okay and what's not.

If you follow this approach, you may be amazed at what your body can do over time. Here's a testimonial from a client who's been practicing the ChiRunning technique for three years.

I have slowly been increasing my distance and have been maintaining my running routine for over a year. I now know that I will be able to run for as long as I want to. Also, I know that someday when I want to try a marathon, I will know what I need to do to train for it. It is amazing how I can actually feel relaxed and energized at the same time while running. In fact, I always feel so much better after running than I did before I went out for a run. Many days I am sluggish and tired, or some part of my body will ache, and I think that I cannot possibly go out and run. But when I start out slowly, with a short stride, I begin to relax all of the tension that has been building in my back and shoulders all day.

From a purely physical viewpoint, ChiRunning can be used to run faster and farther and will definitely make one a better and more relaxed runner. However, I feel that there is so much more to it than that. By practicing the principles of Body Sensing and efficiently using my muscle energy to enjoy my runs, it teaches me that I can learn to sense myself physically and emotionally in all situations and to not waste energy as I journey through life. Incorporating this philosophy with a holistic focus enables me to achieve a true sense of peace and happiness. *Aga Goodsell*

CHAPTER SEVEN

The Beauty of Learning and the Blessing of Challenges

In the middle of difficulty lies opportunity.—ALBERT EINSTEIN

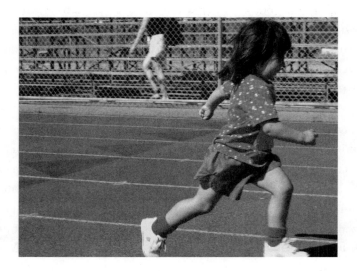

Learning something new is the most powerful way to keep your body and mind vibrant. It's what gives life its spark, and it is what must take place in each of us if we hope to evolve as individuals. With each new undertaking, you'll come up against challenges. In any new venture, you can *expect* new challenges—that's how you grow! Learning is always a stretch, which at times can feel uncomfortable, physically and mentally and emotionally. Use this chapter as a resource to guide you as you meet challenges on the path to improving your running form.

This chapter will address questions and concerns that might arise as you work on your ChiRunning technique. It is a collection of great exercises and form drills designed to give you a clearer sense of what ChiRunning is all about.

THE DIFFERENCE BETWEEN PRODUCTIVE AND NONPRODUCTIVE DISCOMFORT

There's always some discomfort and awkwardness when you learn something new with your body. Do you know anyone who jumped on a bicycle for the first time and pedaled away? Or anyone who stepped on a skateboard for the first time and didn't immediately fall right off? Learning is a process of trial and error, of trying and failing, of getting it and just as easily losing it. When you introduce a new way of moving to your body, the response can sometimes feel wonderful. But many times it takes a period of adjustment before everything moves along smoothly in the new way. During this period of transition, it is important to listen carefully to your body's responses so you can tell whether you're moving correctly. One of the best ways your body has of telling you when you're doing something wrong is by sending your brain messages of discomfort or pain.

If there's any place in our culture where we need healthy change in attitude, it's in our relationship with discomfort and pain. Instead of dealing with discomfort by addressing the cause, we are taught to deny its existence by using painkillers or some other course of symptomatic relief.

Since physical discomfort is a big issue with runners, I want to ease any fears around discomfort by clarifying the difference between productive discomfort and nonproductive discomfort. Productive discomfort leads to progress, while nonproductive discomfort leads to pain and/or injury (figure 86).

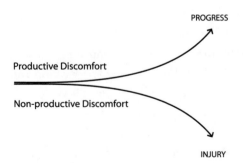

Figure 86—Productive and nonproductive discomfort

Productive discomfort is a necessary part of any growth process. When you start up a running program and get out of breath, it's uncomfortable to feel like you're not getting enough air into your lungs. But it shouldn't come as any surprise that you breathe harder; after all, you're doing something that your body is not used to. If you can make it past the beginning stages, being out of breath will go away in a couple of weeks as your body acclimates to the increased oxygen requirements of running.

Discomfort can be an indicator that you are going beyond your own status quo and feeling the stretch. Here are some everyday examples of productive discomfort:

- Headaches from quitting coffee
- Getting up earlier to exercise
- Eating less to lose weight
- Running in inclement weather
- Lack of sleep with a new baby
- Asking for a pay raise
- Standing in a five-hour line for Rolling Stones tickets

These are all examples of discomforts that are a part of a productive process. Another phrase used to describe productive discomfort was coined by the Russian mystic G. I. Gurdjieff, who called it "intentional suffering," which pretty much tells it like it is.

Nonproductive discomfort is a warning that something is not right with what you are doing, and you need to make an appropriate adjustment or the next sensation you might feel is pain. Pain is your body's way of telling you that you need to be careful not to let your situation degrade into an injury. Discomfort in your knees is an indication that you need to shorten your stride, land more on your midfoot, or correct a pronation problem. Pain is your body's way of telling you to change how you're moving.

In my running career, I have learned the most about running correctly from pain. Whenever I've felt pain, I've had the choice either to

stop running or to run in a way that prevented the pain from occurring. My first impulse has always been to look for the cause, which has
inevitably led to the solution. To make a correction to your running
form, first find out precisely where the sensation is coming from, so
you have a point of reference to start from.

Master Xu tells me that chi is blocked wherever you experience
pain. If you can get into proper alignment, then relax and loosen the
area that is painful, the chi will again flow through the area and help
the pain to subside.

THE BODY SCAN

This is an exercise that you can do anytime you're running. Actually,
you can do it anytime at all, and it will help you to get a clear sense
of the current state of your body. The Body Scan is the gateway to
Body Sensing and will teach you how to communicate with your body.
Good communication is based on an ability to *listen*, whether it's to
your own body or another person. In this exercise you will scan your
body while running and listen for anything needing attention. I also
use the exercise for on-the-run relaxation.

Start at your head and work your way down your body. All you
have to do is focus your attention on each area and see if you sense
any tenseness, stiffness, discomfort, or pain. If you don't, send up a
prayer of thanks and move on. If you feel something that doesn't
seem right, focus your mind on that area and take a deep breath. Try
to relax the area if it's tense or stiff. Move it around or shake it. Let go
of any tension. The pain or discomfort could be from overuse, in
which case you should let it rest and allow another part of your body
to help out.

If you come upon an area that needs lots of work, do a little and
then move on to the rest of your body. When you've relaxed and loos-
ened all the other areas, you can come back to the "biggie" and give it
some special attention.

The following is a sequential list of areas of your body. To familiarize yourself with each of these areas, start at the top of the list. As you
move through, place your hands on each body part. Pause in each lo-

cation for a few seconds and see if you can feel any tension or soreness. Then move on through the list, pausing at each one to listen. If you're reading this book and sitting in a chair, don't get up. You can do this one sitting down.

Touch your...

Head
Neck
Shoulders
Arms
Elbows
Wrists
Hands
Upper back
Chest and breathing
Abdominals
Lower back
Pelvis
Hips
Glutes
Quads
Knees
Calves and shins
Ankles
Feet

When you've finished scanning your whole body, go back and do one last continuous sweep from head to toe, taking about 10 seconds to do it.

TROUBLESHOOTING YOUR CHIRUNNING FORM: COMMON HOT SPOTS

With a good working knowledge of what to do when things don't feel right, you can circumvent the difficulties or discomforts mentioned in the next section. This is a list of the most common concerns that I hear. Following the description of the problem, I'll offer the likely causes. In most cases I will refer you to the form focus most appropriate for your problem.

There is a plethora of books that deal with how to treat the *symptoms* of running injuries, so I won't go into that here. What I will say is that if you can work to correct the *cause* of a problem, it will go away and, in most cases, not recur.

This section is divided into four basic categories within which all form difficulty questions will fall:

Posture
Lean
Upper body
Lower body

Use this section whenever you have an ache or pain associated with your running. The better you are as a detective, the quicker the solution will come.

POSTURE

- **Difficulty sensing what correct posture feels like:** You're not practicing your posture stance enough when you're *not* running, which makes it difficult to feel when you *are* running.

   Spend time practicing your posture while standing still so you can become very familiar with it (see exercise on page 162 and figure 88.) Set aside 10 minutes a day when all you do is stand there, working on straightening your posture, memorizing what it feels like when it's correct. Then, when you're out on your run, you'll be able to recall that feeling.
- **Neck:** Problems with your neck are generally due to your structure not being aligned properly, meaning that you need to work on correcting your posture (see above). Neck pain can also be caused by holding tension there. Be sure to look around while you are running. Don't overfocus on the road or trail directly in front of you. Look up and expand your vision.

LEAN

- **Not feeling your abs working:** If you're not using your abs enough, you won't be able to feel them working. If you're using them correctly, you'll feel like you're doing a crunch. Do the exercise where you lean against a table while keeping your posture straight. This exercise will engage your abs so that the feeling is unmistakable (see figure 22, page 75). Practice often so that you can recall the same feeling in your body when you're running. Be patient and give yourself lots of time to get this. It's completely new territory for most people.

- **Not sensing the forward pull of gravity:** If you don't feel like you're being pulled along by gravity, you're probably not leaning enough. Practice leaning against a wall before you go out for a run. Do it until you come away with a clear Body Sense of what it feels like to fall forward while holding your posture straight. Try to always feel for the sensation in your abdominal muscles, which are doing the work of holding your posture straight and tilted forward. When running, you should always feel the sense of falling forward, even if it's only slight.

UPPER BODY

- **Breathing issues or shortness of breath:** The bottom line is that your muscles are not getting enough oxygen, and here are some possible reasons. Your breath may be too slow or too shallow, which means that your blood is not getting sufficiently oxygenated. You may be running too fast for your current level of conditioning, or using too much muscle. Go to Chapter 3, "Breathing," on pages 51–54.

- **Shoulders:** Many people who complain of tight shoulders tend to run with their shoulders held either too far back or too high. Here are two suggestions:

  1. If you know you hold your shoulders too high, relax them by dangling your arms at your sides for 1 minute, every 15 minutes, while you're running. When you reestablish your arm

swing, bend your arms at a right angle and let your elbows swing freely, keeping your shoulders relaxed and low, just like they were when you were dangling your arms.

2. If you hold your shoulders back, you'll look like the guy in the picture (figure 87). His chin is too high, his shoulders are back, he's bent at the waist, and his posture line looks like a slalom course. This not only puts a strain on your shoulder muscles, it adds extra curvature to your lower back, which can lead to lower-back and neck pain. Go back to Chapter 5 and practice the grounding stance, in "Body Loosening Exercises," on page 108. Body Sense what this feels like and memorize the shape in your shoulders so you can bring it into your running. Every now and then, while you're running, grab the Chi-ball, which will get your back into the correct position.

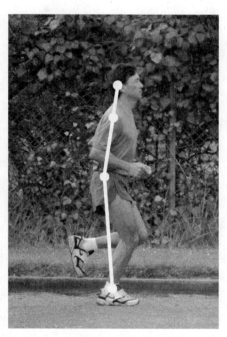

Figure 87—Shoulders back and bent at the waist

LOWER BODY

- **Lower back:** Having tightness or soreness in your lower back can mean that you're bending at the hips as you land on your support leg instead of keeping your posture straight. Bending at the hips forces your lower back muscles to support the weight of your upper body, because it's cantilevered in front of you (figure 87). When you run with straight posture, your structure will support your body weight (figure 88).

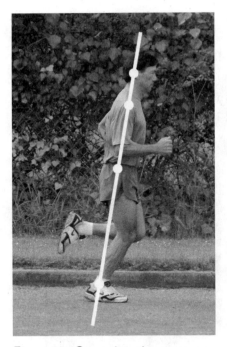

Figure 88—Correct posture: ear, shoulder, hip, and ankle aligned

If you're using your abdominal muscles to support your posture, your back muscles will not be overworked. Shortening your stride length will also take the load off your back. Be sure to keep your cadence between 85 and 90 when you shorten your stride. Here's an exercise for strengthening your abdominal muscles so that your posture is supporting your back instead of your back supporting your posture.

Exercise

This exercise will keep your pelvis level while running, which in turn will prevent bending at the waist. Stand with your feet parallel and hip width apart. Do your basic posture exercise: Straighten your upper spine by holding one hand on your belly button and lifting your collarbone with the other. Now locate your pubic bone and, using your lower abdominal muscles, lift up on it. Don't clench your glutes to tilt your pelvis; just isolate your lower abs to do the job. Here's the final step: Imagine an invisible line running between your pubic bone and your chin (figure 91). Now imagine shortening the length of that line. You'll be dropping your chin and lifting your pubic bone at the same time, shortening the line. This will straighten your neck and level your pelvis, which will flatten your lower back. Practice this in the standing position until you feel familiar with the shape of your spine, then try to integrate it into your running, especially when you're leaning. Your abs will be relieving your lower back muscles of their former duties. Good-bye, back pain.

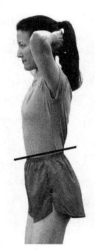

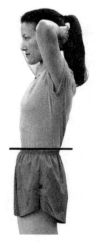

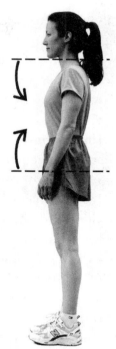

Figure 90—
Abdominals not
lifting (incorrect)

Figure 89—
Abdominals lifting
(correct)

Figure 91—Shorten
the line between
the chin and pubic
bone

- **Hips:** Loosen 'em up, baby! Do hip circles (see page 101) all day, every day, every time you can remember to do them. I had stiff hips, and Master Xilin told me to do 3,000 hip circles—the problem was eradicated in one day.

  You can also practice some extra hip flexor stretches after running (see page 114).

- **Quadriceps:** If your quads are sore, it means you're using them too much. Sorry, overuse is not allowed in ChiRunning. Work your hip flexors instead, and let your quads rest through every phase of your leg swing. Generally, if your quads hurt, it means your foot strike is in front of your body, which increases the impact to your upper legs. Shorten your stride and pull your foot strike back in, more under your body, and you'll reduce the shock to your quads. Picking up your feet will also help reduce shock to your quads, because you'll be creating an upward force to balance some of the downward force of your feet hitting the ground.

The best way to tell if your feet are hitting the ground correctly is if your feet are moving in a rearward direction as they hit the ground.

- **Hamstrings:** If you're experiencing discomfort here, your foot is striking out in front of you, and you're overstriding—pulling yourself forward with each step. This is very hard on your hamstrings. It also happens when you're running uphill and reaching ahead of your body with your legs. Let your lean do the work so your upper body is ahead of where your feet are striking the ground, and the pulling will disappear. Overstriding also means that you are reaching in front of yourself with your stride. Shorten your stride and give your hamstrings a break. Open up your stride *behind* you instead of in front.

- **Glutes:** Loosely translated, this means that you're a tight-ass, just like the rest of us who hold tension here. Work on your control issues—this is not "Buns of Steel" class. Do lots of pelvic circles (see page 102) with your abdominals instead of your glutes. You can also practice relaxing your glutes whenever you're just standing around. I catch myself holding tension here all the time. If you can relax here, you can relax anywhere. It's very subtle but very effective.

- **Knees:** There are many reasons for knee pain. I will list only the most common ones here.

(1) **Foot turnout:** If your feet turn out to the side as you run, it could create knee pain at any distance by torquing your knee with every foot strike (figure 92). This will eventually overwork the ligaments and tendons in the knee and lead to pain and injury. The main reason your foot is turning out is the weak adductor muscles on the inside of your leg. These are the muscles responsible for rotating your legs so that your feet point forward when they land. If you rotate your upper leg inward as you run, it will strengthen

these muscles and eventually relieve the problem. Run like you're on a tightrope, with your feet hitting along a line stretched out along the road in front of you.

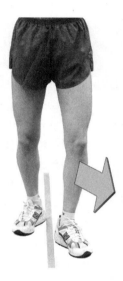 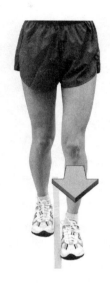

Figure 92—Incorrect   Figure 93—Correct

(2) **Heavy heel strike:** This, in my opinion, is the single most common cause of knee pain. If your feet are striking in front of you, or if you're shuffling, your knees could be taking a lot of abuse (figure 94). Look at it this way. Any time your foot hits the ground in front of your center of gravity, you're momentarily braking because your foot stops while your body continues to move forward. That's why the heels on your shoes wear out—they're like the brake pads on a car. If your foot stops and your body keeps moving, your knee becomes the transfer point for all that force. Well, your knees were designed to be hinges, not shock absorbers, and they get irritated by having to do a task that is not in their job description. So do them a favor and remember to do two things when you run: Pick up your feet with each stride; and run with your upper body in front of your foot strike so that you're landing

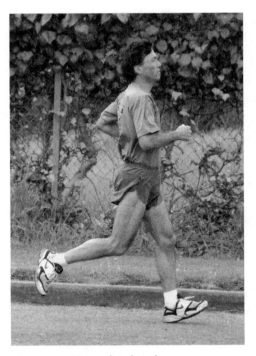

Figure 94—Heavy heel strike

on your midfoot instead of your heel.

(3) **Downhill running:** This section deals with knee pain as related to downhill running. (For a thorough explanation of how to run downhill, see page 178.) On a downhill, there is more pressure on your legs than at any other time in your running. Up to ten times your body weight with each step. This puts a huge demand on your knees and quads. The best way around this is to draw the focus away from your knees and quads by putting your attention on the backs of your legs, which is where your main shock-absorbing muscles are located. Whenever you're running downhill, land with more of your weight on your heels than on your forefoot. If you land on your forefoot, you will engage the front side of your legs (your shins, knees, and quads). If you land on your heels, you will engage the back sides of your legs (your glutes, hamstrings, and calves). Imagine that you have an invisible pole connecting your tailbone and heels, and this invisible pole supports your body weight every time your feet hit the ground. There is a great T'ai Chi stance that will help you develop this sense (see page 182).

Another thing to remember on a downhill is to relax your legs as much as possible. Any extra tension in your legs makes the ride a lot rougher. Pretend you've got limousine shock absorbers instead of the kind used on dirt bikes.

- **Difficulty holding a cadence of 85 to 90 strides per minute:**
  Your stride length is too long for the speed that you are running.
  The three things that will help you get your cadence are: a quicker
  arm swing, a shorter stride, and picking your feet up. These are
  covered in Chapter 4.

  When you work to increase your cadence, do so in very small increments. If you're starting with a cadence of 75 and you want to
  increase it to 85, don't do it all at once. All you have to do is increase
  your cadence by 2 steps per minute each week, and in 5 weeks
  you'll be at your target cadence without your body fighting you the
  whole way.

- **Shins and calves:** If your shins are sore, it's because you're using
  them. You'll need to practice relaxing them. You're probably either
  tensing your ankles or pushing off with your toes instead of picking up your feet with each stride (figure 95). It could also be that
  your stride is too long, which inevitably throws you onto your toes,
  thus overworking your shins. Talk to your calves and ankles. Tell
  them they are just along for the ride. Shake them out often whenever you're standing around. Teach them to relax!

  Keep your legs limp from the knees down. Shorten your stride
  and relax your lower legs. I had a client tell me that he remem-
  bered to keep his lower legs limp by pretending he didn't *have* any
  lower legs. Practice picking up your feet while keeping your legs
  limp from the knees down (see page 168) and practice the Sandpit
  Exercise (see page 171).

  Be sure you are landing on your midfoot (which engages your
  core muscles) and not on the ball of your foot (which engages your
  calves) (figure 96). If your calves are chronically tight, massage
  them often, especially after each run. Work hard at not holding
  tension in your ankles, and take hot baths after workouts.

  If you're recovering from shin splints, be sure to run on flat surfaces. Running up hills will sometimes force you onto your toes,
  which will aggravate your shins and slow your healing process.
  Running with shin splints is an opportune time to learn how to run
  without using your lower legs, because if you can relax them, they

won't hurt. But as soon as there's any tension in your calves, you'll feel it.

Another potential cause of sore calves is not taking in enough water or electrolytes while running, which cramps the calves. This can be very painful and can quickly reduce a run to a walk. Refer to "Muscle Cramps," page 174.

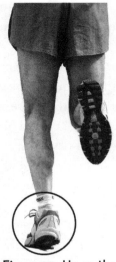

Figure 95—Up on the balls of the feet (incorrect)

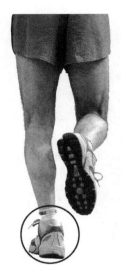

Figure 96—Landing on the midfoot (correct)

- **Heavy or plodding stride:** Your stride is too long, and your emphasis is on the impact of your feet instead of on picking them up. Practice focusing your attention on the foot that is coming up off the ground. Always think of picking up your feet instead of landing. Also practice your posture while running. Keep it elongated while you're leaning.

Exercise: Bending Your Knees

This exercise is the best cure for heavy foot strikers. It will help you pick up your feet *without* picking up your knees (which should always stay low).

Part 1

- Stand with good posture, keeping your Column in mind.
- Hold your arms at your sides with your elbows straight and your hands holding the sides of your legs (figure 97).
- Run in place by keeping your knees down and gently picking up your feet behind you (figure 98). Bend your knee enough to get your shin parallel to the ground (your leg will be bent at a right angle). Do not let yourself bend at the waist or lift your knees (that's why you're holding on to your legs with your hands). You should feel yourself landing on your midfoot, not on your toes (figure 99). You should *not* be pushing off with your toes (which causes you to bounce up and down). It's just a heel lift and a knee bend.

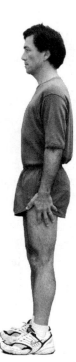

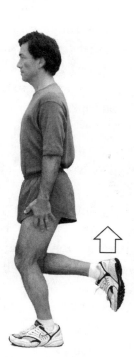

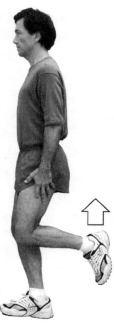

Figure 99—Land on your whole foot

Figure 98—Run in place with knees down, heels up

Figure 97—Bend-knee exercise: hold on to your quads

- Keep your lower legs as limp as you can while doing this exercise. (This includes your toes, feet, ankles, and calves.)
- Run in place for a count of 30 knee bends.
- Stop and rest for 30 seconds.
- Repeat this exercise 3 times and try to get as relaxed as you can while doing it.

Part 2: The Running Version of the Knee-Bending Exercise

- Find a flat place where you can run for at least 100 yards.
- Do the above exercise one more time and recall the body sensation of the previous exercise (relax, pick up your feet, keep your Column straight, hang on to your quads, and bend your knees).
- Now do it again, except this time you'll be adding in a tilt to your Column. Start by running in place. Once you've established running in place, drop your attention to the bottoms of your feet. Keep your feet hitting at the bottom of your Column, then simply let your Column tilt forward slightly. Don't change a thing that you're doing with your body, just add a *slight* tilt (only an inch or two), and remember to lean from your ankles. Feel gravity pull your body forward. Be sure you're not tensing your ankles at all by keeping your lower legs limp.
- Find a spot on the ground about 20 yards from where you are starting. When you pass that point, bend your arms and swing your elbows to the rear (the standard arm swing position). If all goes well, you will feel yourself pulled forward by your lean. Pick up your feet to keep up with your forward momentum. Visualize yourself moving along on a conveyor belt. Do it by feel, and remember, you're teaching your body something new, and you don't have to get it right the first time. Relax and try it again, or as many times as it takes to feel the pull of gravity and the lift of your feet.

It's important to keep your knees down because lifting your knees will bring your foot strike too far forward, into the territory where greater impact and heel striking occur. If you keep your knees down, your feet will strike under or behind your center of gravity, where they need to, and your knees will swing forward without coming up.

- **Difficulty learning how to pick up your feet when running:** If you're having a hard time picking up your feet, this exercise is great, a favorite in all the beginning classes. It's a fun way to learn how to run completely different than you're used to. If you're one of those runners who has a hard time breaking yourself of the habit of overusing your lower legs, you'll learn how *not to push off* with your feet. It's also good practice for running in sand or snow.

The Sandpit Exercise

This exercise is good for learning to pick up your feet and maintain limp lower legs at the same time. Many runners have had remarkable results after doing it only 5 minutes. Practice this *all the time* when you're running.

Find a place to run in the sand. If you live near the coast, this is relatively easy. If you live inland, go to your local high school track and see if there's a broad-jump pit. Level a path in the sand the length of the pit. Start by walking across the sand as if you are walking on thin ice. Pick up your feet with each step and try to leave perfectly flat, crisp footprints; you'll have to relax your ankles to do this. When you can do this, run across the sand at a very slow speed, taking small steps and picking up your feet as you go. Then go back and look at your tracks. Is there a little crater at the front of each footprint? If so, you are pushing off with your toes instead of picking up your feet (figure 100).

Now clean the path again, and run across the sand, letting your lower legs be totally limp while picking up your feet. Have the image in mind that you don't want to disturb the sand as you run across it. You can also pretend you're running across hot coals barefoot. Whatever works . . . When you get good at this exercise, you'll see a nice, clear, undisturbed set of footprints, with no craters (figure 101). When you've practiced enough to leave good footprints in the sand, try to Body Sense what it is you're doing so you can instate all of the same motions into your regular running.

When you are finally able to run the length of the sand without "cratering," do this: At the end of most broad-jump pits is a runway that the broad jumpers use. Start at the end of the pit opposite the runway and run across the sand. When you get to the other side of the pit, continue running as if the runway were made of deep sand. Float across it the same way you floated across the sandpit, and notice how lightly your feet are touching the ground. The memory of this sensation will be your guide for how your feet should feel all the time. In the future, if you feel that your foot strike is a bit heavy, pretend you are running across the sand, trying to leave perfect footprints.

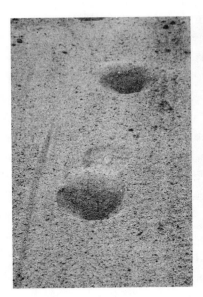 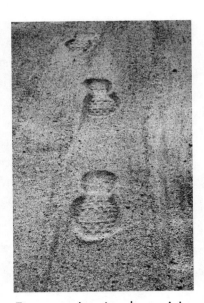

Figure 100—Making craters   **Figure 101—Leaving clean prints**

- **Ankles:** At the risk of sounding repetitive, I'll say it one more time: Most lower leg injuries are from some sort of overuse. If you don't use it, you can't abuse it. Whenever I'm running, I'm always focusing on relaxing my lower legs through every phase of my stride. I try not to use anything below the knee unless I absolutely have to. One of the rare times I use my lower legs is when I'm running on a trail and I come upon lots of gnarly roots that I have to dance over and around. *Then* I'll get up on my toes momentarily to dance around the obstacle. But, as soon as it's passed, I'm back to relaxing my lower legs again.

Another cause of sore ankles is running on roads that have a cant. Most roads and streets are designed with a slight dome along the centerline so water can drain off to the sides. If you're running on the side of a road with a crown, your ankles are constantly landing bent to one side. Switch sides of the road often so that each ankle will be flexed both ways for short but equal periods of time. If you run early in the morning, before the cars are out, you have the luxury of running down the middle of the road, which is generally flat. Just be sure to yield the right of way to anything larger than you.

Another place to watch for a side slope is along a beach. Although it looks great in travel advertisements, it's not the best thing for your ankles, because the sand will always slope toward the ocean. If you really have to run on the beach, just run a short distance, then turn around so your ankles can bend the other way for a bit. Save looking good for the nightclubs.

- **Achilles tendon:** If you're relaxing your lower legs when you run, your Achilles tendon will not be overworked. If you've injured or pulled it, stay off the hills until the soreness is gone. When you add hills back into your program, just make them light and easy at first until your Achilles tendon gets used to the idea. Although you might be tempted, don't stop walking or running when you have an Achilles pull; without some amount of stretching during the healing process, it will heal at a shorter length, leaving you vulnerable to a repeat injury. If it's just too painful to run on, take it easy and run at the first possible opportunity. Ice it often to keep any swelling down. And, once again, *relax* your lower legs when you run. Achilles-tendon pulls are one of the best times to learn how to relax your lower legs. Pool running is a great way to keep your legs in shape while recovering from an Achilles pull.
- **Plantar fasciitis:** This is an injury to be avoided at all costs. It's painful and takes forever to heal because you're always on your feet. If

you have any pain on the soles of your feet between the ball of your foot and your heel, you could be heading into plantar fasciitis territory. When you first feel the symptoms, ice your foot to reduce any inflammation (ideally, hold it in an ice bath for 10 minutes or more if you can stand it), and stay off hills until the soreness goes away. To strengthen your plantar muscle, you can pick up marbles with your toes, or if you've lost your marbles, you can do towel scrunches.

Sometimes plantar fasciitis is an indicator that you're due for new shoes. The midsole of your running shoes breaks down with age, reducing the amount of cushioning, which can cause bruising on the bottoms of your feet.

Plantar soreness can sometimes be mistaken for other foot pains. If you feel pain in your arches, your shoes might be too stiff or laced too tightly.

- **Muscle cramps:** These are caused mostly by dehydration and/or a low level of electrolytes. If your body is low on water or electrolytes, it will have a difficult time conducting the electrical current necessary for the firing of your muscles.

  Here's the preventive thing to do: Drink 12 ounces of water or sports drink a half hour before you exercise. If you'll be out running over an hour, wear a fanny pack and carry your own water or sports drink. Ask fellow runners or your local running store what sports drinks they would recommend. Then test them out on your runs to see how your body adapts to each one. Look for one that is easy to drink, tastes decent, and has an ingredients label that doesn't look like a chemistry final.

  When I'm racing, I set my countdown timer for 10-minute intervals and drink electrolyte-replacement fluid every time it goes off. This keeps me well hydrated, and I never have muscle cramps. I call it the drip system. An alternative to electrolyte replacement drinks is taking electrolyte capsules (not salt tablets). They eliminate the need to carry anything except water. And the best part is that you don't have to drink that nasty stuff they serve at aid stations.

These tips will help you in the early stages of learning the ChiRunning technique. Remember the three P's: practice, perseverance, and patience. If you need additional help, you can always add in two more P's: positive attitude and prayer.

SPECIAL CIRCUMSTANCES

UPHILL RUNNING

There's a lot to be said about running up hills. The main thing is that it brings a third dimension into your running: elevation. There's something very satisfying about cresting a hill and looking back on what you just did. Many people shy away from hills, thinking they're so much more work. But let me clue you in on a little secret—*it's not that much more work*. That is, if you can train your body to do it on technique instead of muscle.

ChiRunning not only makes running easier on flats, it makes running easier on hills. When you're running on a level surface, as I've mentioned, think of your body as a team of two—upper body and lower body—with a shared responsibility of supporting your running. When running uphill you'll need to change this proportion to ensure your legs are not overworking. Your upper body needs to work a little harder on the uphills. So, instead of the balance being 50/50, the new percentages will look more like 60/40 or 70/30. It's not just a matter of increasing your upper body effort; it also means reducing your lower body effort. The best way to reduce your lower body effort is to relax everything below your waist as much as possible. Relaxing your legs shortens your stride length, which shifts you to a lower gear. Isn't that what you do in your car when you go uphill? In order to have good energy efficiency, your body has to follow the same laws of physics that any machine would. So, downshift and use your gears.

Since you're not using your legs as much, you'll have to shift your energy expenditure to your upper body. Swinging your arms and leaning are the ticket. Uphill arm swing should be forward, not to the rear, as in flat running. Keep your hands close to your body and swing in an upward motion, starting from your hips and bringing your hands up to your face. Pretend you're trying to punch yourself in the chin. An upward swing will give your body the upward momentum it needs.

The other important aspect of running uphill is leaning forward into the hill. Here's what happens. When you are running on a level surface, you're tilting forward at an angle to the ground. As the hill comes up in front of you, you may feel thrown back upright by the hill, which causes you to step up the hill in front of your body. This will overwork your hamstrings and lower legs because you're reaching up the hill for your next step. In order to counteract this tendency, *stay forward* and keep your lean working so that your feet land underneath your centerline and not in front of it.

These are the things to remember on the uphills: Shorten your stride, lean forward, swing your arms up to your face, relax your legs, keep your heels down. Relaxing your legs will reduce your perceived exertion level and leave you with the sense that running uphill is not much more difficult than running on a level surface.

- **Steep uphills:** If you like to run hills, you'll eventually find yourself in a situation where you come upon a major hill that seems

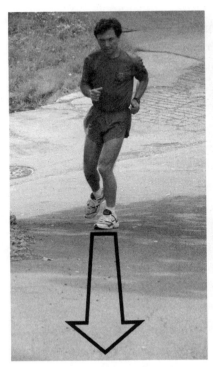 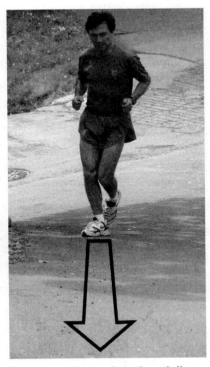

Figure 102—Lateral stride uphill, step 1

Figure 103—Lateral stride uphill, step 2

like a "walker." The reason steep hills are so tiring is that keeping your heels down is difficult. You are forced up onto your toes to prevent your Achilles tendons from being overstretched. Then your calves get tired from doing all the work of keeping you on your toes, so you stop and walk.

There's a way around this scenario: sideways. That's right, turn your hips to one side and run up the hill sideways. Your feet will be doing a little crossover step, but your heels will be down, meaning that your Achilles tendons will not be overstretched and your calves won't be overworked (figures 102–104). I call it the *lateral stride*. The beauty of this unconventional technique is that it engages your lateral muscles (side of the leg). These muscles are generally not used much when you're on level ground, so it's like having a fresh set of muscles helping you out. When I start up a steep hill, I'll run with my body turned about 45 degrees to one side for 6 to 8 strides, then switch sides. In this way, I allow my lateral leg muscles to alternate between running and resting by working one set of muscles and then the other.

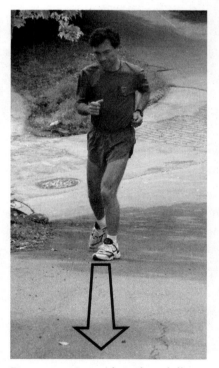

Figure 104—Lateral stride uphill, step 3

Your arm swing will also be different on steep uphills. When you turn your body to one side, your uphill arm will swing sideways relative to the slope of the hill, rendering it pretty useless. Don't worry about it. Just let it swing lightly and don't put a whole lot of work into it. On the other hand (no pun intended), your downhill arm is aiming in the uphill direction, so let it swing fully across your body, reaching up for your opposite shoulder. Shorten your stride. Remember, it's a steep hill, so shift to an even smaller gear. And lean in to the hill with your uphill shoulder—as if you're trying to break down a door. Hey, whatever image works . . .

I've heard many giggles from running-class participants when I mention going uphill sideways—until they try it. Then those giggles turn to laughter when they see how easy it is to run this way up a steep hill. I've even had clients say that it was the single most important thing they learned, because they no longer have to limit themselves to flat running. That alone is worth it.

DOWNHILL RUNNING

The key to comfortable, smooth downhill running is knowing how to relax, both physically and mentally. If you tense your muscles on the way down a hill, you'll jar your legs more than is necessary and wear yourself out more quickly. Learning how to mentally relax while running downhill is really the more difficult aspect, because for many people, it is when they are running at their fastest speed.

The main focus is on lowering the impact to your legs and back so you can arrive at the bottom in much the same condition as when you left the top. For me, running downhill can be the most joyful part of a workout. I imagine myself flowing down the hillside like a stream seeking the quickest course. It's a time when I can relax and surrender, and let gravity take over.

I split downhill running into two categories—runnable and nonrunnable. Some hills are so gradual that you don't have to put on the brakes. Those are the ones I call *runnable*. It's a time to loosen your hips, stretch out your stride, and let gravity do the work. On this type of hill, you can learn how to soften your body, relax, and take it easy while running at speeds you normally only dream of. Then there are the steeper hills, where you spend most of your time slowing yourself down so things don't get out of control. These I call *nonrunnable* hills.

- **Runnable downhills:** Here is a list of focuses that will help you experience new levels of speed and looseness on those easy downhills.

- Relax your mind and surrender to the speed, Grasshopper.
- Relax everything from the waist down, and pay special attention to relaxing your quads and calves.
- Lean downhill and keep your upper body ahead of your foot strike.
- Relax your lower back by letting your pelvis rotate from side to side. Every time your leg swings out the back, let your hip be pulled back with it. This will help your pelvis learn to rotate. Your pelvic rotation will allow your stride to open up behind as you run downhill. With each stride, keep your foot on the ground as long as you can. If you can hesitate for a split second before you pick up your foot, you'll begin to feel your hip bones pulled back by your legs as your stride opens up behind you.
- Do a vertical crunch. Many runners pull their shoulders back when running downhill. This puts more curve into your lower back, increases the pressure on your sacrum, and throws your legs too far forward, which makes you land hard on your heels. If you hold your body in a crunch position (pelvis tilted up in front, shoulders rounded slightly forward), it will flatten your lower back and reduce the impact to your sacrum. When you hold the Chi-ball, your shoulders are slightly rounded forward, which keeps your lower back flat. Practice this stance when you're not running so you can instate it when you're heading downhill.

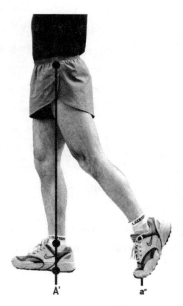

Figure 105—Neutral position: no twist in the spine

Exercise: The Twist-and-Tilt

This exercise will train your hips and sacrum to relax so that your stride can lengthen as you pick up speed on the downhills.

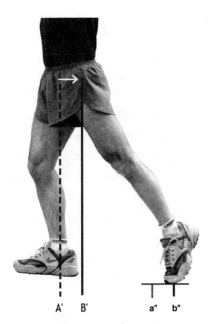

Figure 106—As your hip swings to the rear, your stride lengthens

A'   B'   a"   b"

Every time your leg goes out behind you, let your hip be pulled along with it. This will allow your pelvis to rotate back and forth, causing a slight twist along your spine. Watch for that twist. It means you're doing the right thing—relaxing your lower back and rotating your pelvis more. It happens because your hips are rotating counter to your shoulders.

You can do this at any speed. The faster you run, the more relaxed you'll need to be from the waist down. Relaxing your hips and pelvis will increase your stride length about 3 to 5 inches per stride.

The first figure shows the hips in a neutral position with the leg reaching to the rear (figure 105). The position of the hip is *A*, and the place where the toe meets the ground is *a*.

The second figure shows the hip swinging to the rear along with the leg (figure 106). So, the new position of the hip is *B*, and the new position of the toe is *b*, showing the increase in stride length of about 3 inches. Relaxing your lower back allows your spine to twist, which in turn increases the rotation of your pelvis . . . which then allows your speed to increase . . . with *no* additional effort.

- **Nonrunnable downhills:** Here is a list of focuses that will make those steep downhills fun and relaxing.

  - When your car goes down a steep hill, you let up on the gas pedal, right? So, if your lean is your gas pedal, then let it return to vertical on the steep downhills.

- Take smaller steps and focus on picking up your feet with each step instead of coming down on them with your whole weight. This focus alone will significantly reduce the amount of perceived impact to your quads and feet. If you want to run downhill faster, simply pick up your feet faster, and it won't increase the impact to your legs.
- Zigzag down the hill if there's enough room. This will allow your lateral muscles to do some of the shock absorption.
- Relax your shoulders and keep them low. If you need stability, hold your hands out away from your sides. But don't just relax your *shoulders* when you're running down a steep hill. The more you can relax your *whole body*, especially your legs, the softer the trip down will be.
- Let your weight ride softly on your heels, and use the backs of your legs for shock absorption. Stay off your toes (figure 107).

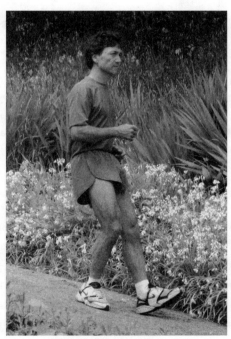

Figure 107—Posture vertical, tailbone tucked, weight on heels

Exercise

Here's a T'ai Chi stance to strengthen your legs for the down-hills. Begin in a grounding stance (figure 108). Then stand with one leg in front of the other (figure 109). All of your weight

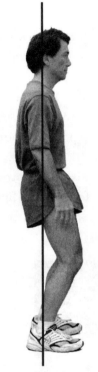

Figure 108—Grounding stance

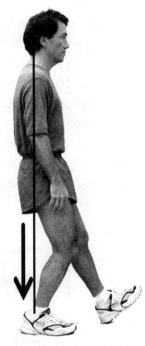

Figure 109—Shift weight to one leg, drop tailbone to heel

should be on the leg under your body. Bend your knee slightly, keeping a straight vertical line between your ear, shoulder, hip, and ankle. Keep your forward leg relaxed, with your heel resting on the ground but not supporting your weight. Stand this way every day for 1 to 2 minutes on each leg. Pretend you have an invisible support leg running from your heel to your tailbone. As your legs become stronger, you'll be able to handle more time on each leg. This is the single most effective exercise that has helped me to improve my downhill running speed and reduced the impact to my quads.

RUNNING IN NEW TERRAIN AND ENVIRONMENTS

Whenever you find yourself running on a different surface than you're used to, or in a different environment, be conscious of all the changes that it might put your body through. If what you're doing is not in your regular program, treat it as an upgrade, which means you'll need to cut back on duration and intensity until your body acclimates to the new conditions. I recommend easing off 15 to 20% on distance, and Body Sensing how much to moderate the intensity. If you're in Hawaii on vacation, you wouldn't want to run the same pace or distance on the beach that you do on the roads at home. Cut back and let your body adjust slowly to the nuances of the new terrain. Your vacation will be much more enjoyable if you're healthy.

If you're thinking of permanently adding a new type of terrain to your running program, do so slowly, in little bits. If you're adding trail running to your program and you've never been on trails, just incorporate a little near the end of your normal run. Then slowly build up the amount each week until you can eventually do the whole run on trails. Whenever you're in doubt about how much to add, just remember the principle of Gradual Progress, and Body Sense what feels like the right amount.

FATIGUE

There are a number of things you can do when you get tired on a run. Just because you're feeling tired doesn't necessarily mean you're at your physical limit. You could be doing something that is causing you to work harder than you need to.

I remember being at mile 80 in the Western States 100 Mile Endurance Run and feeling no energy left in my body. I wasn't sure how I was going to negotiate the last 20 miles, to make my goal of finishing in under 24 hours. I stopped at an aid station and picked up my pacer (in some ultras, you are allowed to have someone run with you after the halfway point), Antoinette Addison, whom I had been coaching for two years. She knew all the form focuses like the back of her hand and kept repeating them to me constantly all the way until the end of the race. Once I started engaging the focuses, I began to regain some of my mental and physical strength. Enough, in fact, to make those last 20 miles the fastest of my entire race! Where did that energy come from? As I've said before, if you set up the right conditions, your chi will flow. As long as I had the strength to keep my form in good shape, I had the energy to run. Whenever I lapsed or lost my focus, I'd have to stop and walk, which was costing me valuable minutes. Antoinette's mission was to keep my mind working by engaging me with focuses. When *that* was happening, I could keep myself running. Because of her constant reminders, I was able to finish a scant 7 minutes ahead of my target time of 24 hours.

When you get tired, your form generally starts to fall apart, which in turn uses even more energy. Here are some focuses to remember when you're feeling tired:

- Shorten your stride.
- Correct your posture. Make sure your feet are hitting behind your upper body, not in front of it.
- Engage your lean again, but don't bend at the waist.
- Slow down your pace until you recover some strength.
- Breathe more from your abdomen and increase your breath rate. Some people get tired from breathing too slowly.
- Look up and take in the world around you. Don't focus on your fatigue, or you'll get more tired. Look around and take in energy from the scenery.
- Relax your shoulders. Let your arms dangle at your sides for 30 seconds every 2 miles.
- Pick up your heels and get your feet moving in a circular motion. Stay away from a shuffle.
- Try to relax any muscles that feel particularly tired or sore. This will help keep energy flowing to overworked areas.

It amazes me how tired I can *get* just thinking about how tired I *am*. On the other hand, it amazes me how much more my body can do when it is aligned and relaxed.

ILLNESS AND RUNNING

I don't run when I have a fever, when I'm in the contagious stage of a cold, or when I'm sick and the temperature is below freezing. But otherwise, I'm out there, because it gets my heart pumping, my lungs expanding, and my lymphatic system circulating, not to mention my chi flowing. Again, if you can Body Sense what you need, you'll do fine.

BUYING SHOES

- **How to tell when you need new shoes:** When you take a new pair of running shoes out of the box, write the date on the rear of the shoe with a permanent marker. After you've been running on that pair of shoes for 4 months, see if you sense any stress in your legs (above and beyond the normal) during or after your runs. If the pavement feels a little bit harder or the trails are wearing your legs out more than usual, switch to a new pair of shoes. If those sensations go away with the first run in the new shoes, you've made a good choice. If nothing changes, go back and read Chapter 4. If you log your miles, you should switch shoes after about 500 miles. That number will increase as your running gets smoother and more fluid. I have gotten as much as 750 miles on a pair of racing flats, but that's more the exception than the rule.

- **How to pick the right shoes:** Here's a brief guide to buying running shoes. When you go shopping, you'll be judging the shoes on three criteria: comfort, flexibility, and weight, in that order.

(1) First and foremost, choose a shoe that is comfortable. It should fit like a glove, with no sense of cramping in the toe box. Go to your local friendly running store and ask the salesperson to bring you a shoe in your size that is flexible and lightweight. No clunkers here. Try them all on to see how they fit. You're looking for a shoe that has plenty of room for your toes. They should never be touch-

ing the inside front of the shoe, and your feet should not feel squeezed at all. The closer you can get to bedroom slippers, the better.

(2) The next thing you're looking for is flexibility. Hold the shoe with one hand on the front and the other hand on the heel, and bend it in the same motion it would bend as you run (see figure 110). Watch carefully for where it bends. If it's a good shoe, it will bend right at the ball area (just aft of the toebox). If it bends in the middle, that will overstretch the muscles on the bottom of your foot. If it doesn't bend and feels rather stiff over the length of the sole, forget it. A shoe that doesn't flex well will throw you onto your toes, causing your calves to overwork as you roll

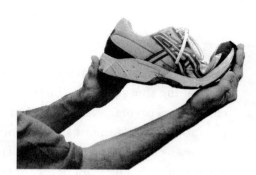

Figure 110—Flexing the shoe

forward off your foot at the end of your stride. No thank you.

(3) Look for a shoe that has some cushioning but is lightweight. Some shoe stores keep a scale on hand. If the shoes weigh in over 14 ounces for a medium-size foot, forget it; you're not looking for combat boots. A good training flat should weigh in under 11 ounces and preferably 8 to 9. Generally speaking, the more a shoe weighs, the stiffer it is, so ask for racing flats or training flats. If you've just started your ChiRunning program and are used to lots of support from your shoes, you can slowly transition into softer and lighter shoes as your form improves. A more neutral shoe trains your foot to do what is necessary for your running, instead of relying on the shoe to do all the work.

Once I went into Chinatown in San Francisco to buy a pair of T'ai Chi shoes. When I told the Chinese woman behind the counter what I wanted, she took one look at the running shoes I had on and said, "I don't understand why Americans wear shoes like *that* . . . all they do is make your feet stupid." What she was implying, in a not too subtle way, was the less shoe you have on your foot, the more your foot will educate your body to move correctly.

For example, people who run barefoot as a rule have much better running form than people who wear shoes. Go to your local track sometime and run a lap without your shoes on, and see what happens to your running form. You'll come back a nonheel striker. Running barefoot forces you to land on that nice, soft midsection of your foot instead of your heel. It also forces you to lean forward, keeping your weight in front of where your feet strike the ground. This is an example of your feet teaching your body how to run correctly. Less is better.

If you find a pair of shoes that really work well for you, go for it and buy as many as 3 or 4 pairs if your budget can handle it. And you can rest assured they won't be around in six months. Finding a good shoe is like finding an honest mechanic—when it happens, it's like striking gold.

If you're a trail runner, you'll need a shoe with an aggressive sole, meaning that it has lugs to improve traction on dirt surfaces. But be careful; shoes that are labeled "trail shoes" are generally pretty stiff and overbuilt. Look for a pair that allows your foot to ride somewhat low to the ground and has a slightly more snug fit so your foot isn't slipping around in the shoe with all the lateral motion of trail running.

- **Breaking in a pair of running shoes:** When you buy a new pair of running shoes, take some time to break them in; don't just throw them on and take off on your long run. Let your body adjust to the new shoes, and let the shoes adjust to you. New shoes, fresh out of the box, will be a little stiff at first, so be aware of what this stiffness can do to your feet and legs: It could cause the muscles in your feet to work harder than they're used to, resulting in some minor muscular irritation or soreness. Follow the principle of

Gradual Progress and take it slowly. Don't do more than about 3 miles on your first outing. After that, the general rule that I follow is not to run over twice the distance of my last run on the new pair. For instance, if your last run on the new shoes was 3 miles, you shouldn't go over 6 miles on the next run.

TREADMILL RUNNING

This section is for those of you who live and run in the northern latitudes, where snow and freezing temperatures often have a big influence on your running program. It's also for those of you who choose to run on a treadmill. (I've always gravitated toward outdoors because there's more chi outdoors than indoors.)

Let me start off by saying that treadmill running is not at all like running on solid ground. It's less of a workout, because the machine is doing the bulk of the work. Also, since the platform is moving, you need to use more ankle muscles for stability with each footstep. If you're doing the ChiRunning technique, you're leaning and lifting. But there is a much higher rate of impact to the knee on a treadmill, because the track is moving toward you. If you're not picking up your feet and leaning enough, a lot of impact is distributed to your legs.

It's also difficult to lean on a treadmill, because there is a tendency to crowd the bar at the front of the machine. I get the jitters running at the back of the treadmill. I feel like any minute I could become a human cannonball and get launched into the wall behind me.

- Begin by setting the speed at a slow enough pace that you can comfortably jog while instating the ChiRunning focuses: posture, lean, picking up your feet, and cadence.
- If you have a treadmill that allows you to run at an incline, tilt it up to the point where you can feel the incline but it's no problem to keep your heels down when landing.
- Most treadmills have a timer on the display panel. Use the seconds counter for setting up your cadence. Every three steps another second should elapse. If that's the case, then your cadence is exactly 90 strides per minute. A cadence of 90 will mitigate the impact of the treadmill on your knees by ensuring that your stride is short.

Another way to keep the impact low is to pick up your feet and move them in a circular path, like a wheel.

- When I tested ChiRunning on a treadmill, I found that speeds faster than a 7-minute mile pace created a lot of impact on my knees that felt unavoidable no matter how much I compensated by leaning. The impact was reduced when I tilted the machine to simulate running up a hill.
- The two things most crucial to good injury-free treadmill running are keeping your stride short and picking up your feet.

MISCELLANEOUS TIPS YOU'LL NEVER FIND IN ANOTHER BOOK

- **Keeping your shoes tied:** How many times have you double-knotted your laces to keep them from coming untied only to be unable to adjust them in the midst of a run because of cold fingers? If you're tired of your shoes coming untied, here are two ways to eliminate the problem forever.

(1) After making the first loop with your laces, wrap the other lace around the loop *twice* instead of once, then finish tying the bow. If you want to untie your shoes, simply pull on the lace ends and . . . ta-da!

(2) Tie your shoes in a regular bow and then take both loops, hold them together, and tuck them under one of the laces farther down on the shoe. My shoes have *never* come untied with this one, and it also keeps my loops from getting caught on branches, which is a real drag. This method also allows you to untie the laces with a simple pull.

- **Drinking from a paper cup at an aid station:** Have you ever grabbed a paper cup at an aid station in a race and spilled half of it before it reached your mouth? Try this. Grab the cup and, after thanking the volunteer who handed it to you, crimp the top so the only opening is a little spout between your thumb and forefinger. Hold the rest of the cup closed with your fingers and the heel of your hand. No slop!

- **How to deal with powdered electrolyte drinks during a race:** If you prefer powdered electrolyte-replacement drink, you'll love this one. Buy a couple of Gel Flasks (made by Ultimate Designs) at your local running store. They're small plastic pop-top bottles that hold only about 3 or 4 ounces. If you're using a scoop of powder per water bottle you can get four bottles' worth of electrolyte replacement into each flask by mixing up a concentrated slurry of powder and warm water. Fill the flask halfway and pour in four scoops of powder (I mix mine with a chopstick). Keep your flask in your water belt. When you need a refill of electrolyte drink, just run through the next aid station with the top off your bottle and ask a volunteer to pour water into your bottle. When it's near full, take out your handy-dandy flask and give it a squirt, and you're outta there in no time, with no sticky fingers.

- **Running and racing in extremely hot conditions:** If you're racing on a very hot day, check to see if the aid stations will have ice. Wear a hat with a brim, and if you can get ice, grab a few cubes and stick them in the top of your hat. You might need to tighten the brim so they won't fall out. As the ice slowly melts, it will keep your head cool, which, by the way, is crucial if you want to keep your brain working well. Heat exhaustion can strike when your brain's temperature rises even a small amount.

  If there isn't any ice available, soak a handkerchief and keep it on your head.

- **Poison oak and poison ivy:** Wash your body in dish detergent immediately after a run where you suspected that you might have come in contact with either one. The rash is spread by oils on the leaves, so a good detergent will cut the oil and wash away the danger.

- **How to stay hydrated without having to stop and pee:** If you have a countdown timer (which I highly recommend), set it to beep every 10 minutes and take a sip every time it goes off, *no matter what.* It helps to carry a water bottle with an electrolyte replacement. This will also be a major factor in whether or not your legs cramp up on you.

- **Running form check-in:** When your beeper goes off, also check on your form. Are you tight anywhere? Are you overworking any muscles, landing too heavy, not lifting your legs? Are you relaxing your breath and smiling?
- **Fatigue:** If you're tired, the two most important things you can do are shorten your stride length and lean more.

CHAPTER EIGHT

Peak Performance and Racing

Trying to do well and trying to beat others are two different things. Excellence and victory are conceptually distinct . . . and are experienced differently.—ALFIE KOHN

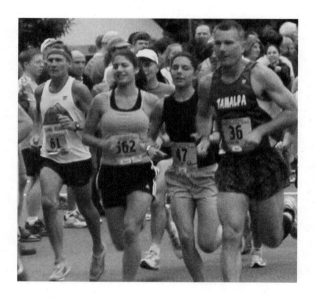

M ost people think that a peak performance just happens, created by some invisible power. Sometimes it does happen that way—by grace. But you can have these experiences on a regular basis in your running, your racing, and your life, if you set up the right conditions. It doesn't need to be a haphazard occurrence.

Peak performance is not about racing, it's about having a clear vision of how you'd like to improve yourself, then setting a goal that embodies the vision, learning and practicing, and training your body to move in the direction of your vision. When the time is right, throw yourself into a single event as a means to acknowledge what you've done and to learn what still needs some attention. A peak performance might be planned out over a six-month period, or it might happen spontaneously one day during a casual workout. It happens when you bring all that you are capable of into the activity before you and sustain it throughout. A peak performance isn't measured solely in results. It's measured internally *and* externally. It's how you feel before, during, and after an event, combined with the results.

When you have a peak performance, you feel yourself moving with the flow of Nature. You're in harmony with what you are supposed to be doing and you're set up to be a conduit for the flow of chi. It's when you finish an event knowing that you've given it your best shot, doing all you were capable of. In these terms, a peak performance might not even be your fastest performance.

The venue for a peak performance is dictated by your level of conditioning and expertise. You wouldn't try for a peak performance on a 10K run if your goal is to run a good 5K. Likewise, you wouldn't go for a peak performance on a hilly course if you haven't done any hills in practice. A peak performance is when you accomplish what you have set out to do, and it is *rarely* an accident. It's intentional from the time you start your first training workout to the last stride of your event.

The key phrase at work here is "striving for something beyond your current level of experience." You could be a first-time runner attempting to run a 12-minute mile or a seasoned runner aiming to finish your first marathon. It's all relative.

RACING

I love to race, mostly because it's the perfect opportunity to practice being present for an extended period of time. I love not only the race but the training and the planning and the strategizing. Racing, to me, is like a final exam to see how well I did my "homework" and whether or not all of my "studies" will pay off. A good day is when I finish well compared to my past performances. If I finish ahead of others in my age group, that's icing on the cake but not the goal. I can have a peak performance no matter who finishes ahead of me.

Whenever I mention racing in my classes, people come back with statements like "I'm too old, too slow, too uncoordinated." To which I respond that racing is the perfect opportunity to have a peak performance, and it could happen for anybody, at any level of skill or conditioning. You don't have to be a hotshot to have a peak performance. All it requires is that you put everything you know into what you are doing. Striving for a peak performance is an opportunity to see yourself really differently. It all comes back to setting up the right conditions, and then magic happens.

"This is only a test . . ." That familiar radio line lets us know that our dashboard will soon be emitting a screech that sounds like an owl in distress. But I like to use it to describe racing: It is only a test.

Performance anxiety brings up a lot of fears around racing. The best way to manage the associated stress is to eliminate it, which means studying your subject until it's as familiar as that face you see in the mirror each morning. This chapter is about how to train smart so you can run smart. Peak performance is not about muscle, it's about mind. You don't have to race to strive for a peak performance, but it does bring out the best in people who approach it with the right attitude. Peak performance is not about racing as much as it's about doing something well, thoroughly, with intention, with finesse—doing the best you can do.

I'll use racing as a metaphor for preparing for a peak performance. Here's how I prepare for and run races so that I can come away with the most. Everything I do to run a race well, I also do for a peak performance. Here are the areas to pay attention to:

- **Your technique:** Have a good working knowledge of the ChiRunning focuses and how to apply them. Constantly work to perfect your technique, especially in the areas where you feel the weakest.
- **Your training:** Develop and plan a personally tailored program: daily, weekly, monthly. Have a good attitude about your program and exhibit perseverance with your training. Know what you need to do to get yourself from where you're starting to the day of your race in the best possible condition, physically and mentally.
- **Your event:** Have a clear logistical plan of what you intend to do on race day, along with a strategy for using everything that you have been practicing.

Race-Specific Training

I was always a lousy test-taker in school. Aside from having poor study habits, I never learned how to figure out what would be required of me on test day. I had friends who seemed to barely study and ace every test. When I'd ask them how they did it, they would usually reply, "I just figured out what I thought they were going to ask and studied that. Then I just glossed over the rest." Easy for you to say.

The only real tests I take now are every three years so I can qualify to sit behind the wheel of an automobile. But another type of test I take is on race day. A race is a physical version of an exam. It's there to measure how well you prepared yourself and how well you work your way through all the problems that are presented. I *have* learned, over all my years of racing, how to do well on this type of test. This chapter is devoted to some of the tricks I've picked up along the way.

How would you like to run a peak performance in your next race? Whether you're a seasoned veteran of many races, or it's your first race, you can optimize your chances by doing some homework in the weeks leading up to the race.

It is no surprise that many races (those not large enough to attract the Kenyans) are won by locals. You can call it the home-field advantage, but what does that mean? Quite simply, that the locals get to practice on the course and familiarize themselves with all the nuances of the layout. They know when they can afford to rest, when to push the pace, and how to adjust their effort level with all of the little demands that the course will throw at them. The smart runners know what to expect and train accordingly. Regardless of the distance, race-specific training gives you a huge advantage, whether you're trying to beat the competition or go for a PR.

What is race-specific training? It's gearing your training toward the specific challenges of an event. Training this way will prepare you better for anything that may come up on race day. Is the course hilly or flat? Will there be aid stations? Is it on trails, asphalt, or concrete? Will weather be a factor? Will the start be crowded? Answering these questions will give you a clearer sense of how to train yourself to be ready for *anything* when race day comes. Nobody likes to be blind-sided, especially in a race.

A little planning goes a long way, but it's best to start your race-specific training a couple of months before the race. This will be in *addition* to whatever you normally do to condition yourself.

First, find a race within the parameters of what you'd like to train for. Many have websites offering all the information you'll need. If it isn't in your vicinity, write or e-mail the race director for a map and an elevation profile. Or try to find people who have done the race in the past and pick their brain for all the details. Drive the course, if it's in your vicinity, or better yet, run it. Then make notes of what the course is like, mile by mile. Here are some of the questions you might ask yourself, along with some suggestions for how to launch your race-specific training program.

Every race-specific training program is designed around three factors: terrain, logistics, and personal experience.

TERRAIN

- What is the first mile of the race like—flat, uphill, or downhill?

  Start your training runs with a first mile similar to the first mile of the race. About two weeks before the race, practice starting slower than your projected average race pace. I mark off the first mile in quarter-mile increments with duct tape so I can practice at my projected starting pace. In this way I can make small adjustments to my pace every quarter mile, instead of running a mile and then realizing I'm way off pace. (I restrict my markings to roads, and I never mark tracks or bike paths.)

- What is the running surface like? Does it change during the course?

  Do some of your training runs on the same surface. I've met many runners who trained for a marathon on trails and then got hammered when they went to race a road marathon.

- Are there any hills? If so, how long and how steep are they? At what miles do the hills appear?

  Add hills to at least one of your weekly runs—preferably of the same height and grade—and/or substitute hill intervals for track workouts. The goal of a successful hill runner is to hold a comfortable pace without getting tired legs. It's a great place to practice technique.

Be sure to add hills at the same points they will appear in the race. If there is a significant hill 3 miles into a race, throw a significant hill 3 miles into your training runs. Be creative and design a race course mock-up in your area so you can go out and do weekly training runs on it.

- Is the altitude of the race course higher than where you normally train?

If it's a significantly higher altitude, do some acclimation runs within two weeks of the actual race. If you don't live within driving distance of high-altitude running, you can help yourself out by practicing your belly-breathing technique during training runs to increase your oxygen intake. If the race is at a lower altitude, thank your lucky stars and have fun.

LOGISTICS

- How often do aid stations appear, and what will they be stocked with?

Never eat or drink something in a race that you haven't tried out on your body beforehand. Who knows, you might be allergic to whatever sports drink they offer. If aid stations are too spread out for your needs, carry your own fluid supply. If you plan to drink the provided sports drink, try it during a training run to see if it works for you.

- How big is the race—hundreds or thousands of people?

If you're going for a PR, don't pick a crowded race and make sure you start toward the front of the pack.

- What time of day does the race start?

Within two weeks of the race date, begin most of your training runs at that time.

- Will you be running the race with friends, or maybe just starting the race with friends?

Be diligent about practicing your starting pace (slower than what you expect to average), and don't get swept into someone else's.

- What is your hydration plan?

  If it's a warm climate, practice hydrating. Know your limits and how much water and electrolyte replacement your body requires. Everybody is different. I've learned that if I drink a mouthful of water every 10 minutes, I don't get dehydrated or have to stop and pee. Long training runs are a good time to find out your body's tolerances. If your sports watch has a countdown timer, use it to time your drinking intervals and see what works for you.

- What is your electrolyte-replacement plan?

  After much trial and error, I've stuck with using electrolyte capsules, available online. Look for vendors who serve the endurance-athlete community or in some drugstores. The capsules are convenient and take the worry out of running a race where you don't know what's being served at the aid stations. I take one every hour, and they always keep me from getting muscle cramps.

PERSONAL EXPERIENCE

- Have you run the distance before this race?

  It is a great physical *and* psychological advantage to run the race distance ahead of time so you know what your body will go through. Race day is not the best time to be going into frontierland.

- How many weeks are there before the race?

  Leave plenty of time to ramp up, train, and taper so you are in your best shape on race day. Two months before you race, adjust your regular training to include race-specific training.

- Do you have any other physical events close to the day of the race?

  Cancel them if this race means a lot to you. I've seen people ruin a race by doing something as innocent as gardening the day before. Plan to take off the day before. If you're traveling there, get there early, set yourself up, and then chill.

GREAT TRAINING TIPS

In addition to all of the above questions, here are some helpful guidelines for what to do during your race-specific training.

- **Hydration:** Practice drinking water while running. Drink electrolyte-replacement drinks before and during your workouts. This will help to replace the minerals that your body loses when you sweat. You should drink 2 to 4 ounces of water for each 15 to 20 minutes of running or walking on your training runs and during the race itself. Hydrate well before and during the race. Drink 12 to 20 ounces of water at least 2 hours before the race.
- **Training diet:** Always eat a good protein meal (meat, fish, poultry, tofu) after a strenuous workout. It helps your body build muscle tissue. Eat a carbohydrate meal (whole-wheat bread, whole grains, whole-wheat pasta, and starchy vegetables) the night before any workout you consider physically challenging. Likewise, try to avoid the heavier protein meals before a hard workout. (This topic is covered more thoroughly in Chapter 9.)
- **Pre-race diet:** Days 6, 5, and 4 before the race, eat protein for breakfast and dinner (soy products, meat, fish, or beans and rice). Days 3, 2, and 1 before the race, eat only carbohydrates (no protein), like whole-wheat pasta (use meatless sauce), whole grains, and veggies.
- **Race day:** Eat foods that digest quickly, providing blood sugar. Eat lightly—bananas, toast and honey, fruits, dates or raisins—and don't eat anything you're not used to.
- **Post-race diet:** A good protein meal (meat, fish, poultry, tofu) after a race helps your body rebuild muscle tissue. It's also important to replace minerals by eating leafy green salads and vegetables soon after the race.
- **Shoes:** If you're planning to get new shoes for the race, buy and wear them at least three weeks before the race, *not* the same week! Most shoes tend to be stiff right out of the box, and you could get blisters from wearing shoes that aren't broken in yet.
- **Starting pace:** Practice your starting pace. Don't go out too fast! Most people start out too fast and burn out after a mile or two. Start at what you consider to be a good medium pace. If your muscles are burning, you're going too fast. Stay relaxed, and you'll do much better.

Go out and mark a 1-mile section of road which mimics the first mile of your race. Practice running a mile at a pace that's 30 seconds *slower* than your projected average pace per mile for the race. This will be your starting pace. Learn what it feels like in your body and remember it on race day.

- **Taper:** Taper off your training two weeks before the race, with no building or speed work. Don't do *slower* runs; just do *shorter* runs at the same pace you would normally train at. It's best to keep your legs sharp but rested.

- **Easy/hard:** Each week alternate easy runs with harder runs, so there'll be no danger of overtraining. If you do hills one day, do flat the next day. If you do speed work one day, follow it with an easy run.

- **If your race is hilly:** Practice running hills by doing short hill intervals. These should be 1 to 2 minutes of uphill running followed by 1 to $1^1/2$ minutes of downhill. Start off easy, and gradually build in intensity and speed with each interval. Be sure to warm up well before a hill workout. Do at least 2 miles of flat running before heading up. This will help to prevent muscle pulls due to cold muscles.

- **Train with a buddy:** Find a training partner and use each other as inspiration to stay with your individual programs. You can also help each other by critiquing each other's running form.

- **Endurance training:** If you're training to do a 5K or 10K, build up to where you can do at least one 5K or 10K per week in training. You marathoners should be trained to run 26.2 miles on a moment's notice. Training your body for endurance is the best guarantee that you'll have a good run on race day.

  Try to vary your weekly training runs so everything you'll need will be built in to your body by race day.

- **Race-course familiarity:** Get a map and drive or run all sections of the course so you know what to expect and where to expect it.

- **Resting on the run:** If you get tired during a run, relax your whole body and lean forward from your ankles up. Let gravity do the work, and let your legs rest.

- **Asphalt running:** When you're out on your training runs, imagine yourself running on thin ice, and that will train you to run with a soft foot strike. If your race is on paved roads, do the majority of your training runs on pavement.

RACE-DAY TIPS

Here's a list of reminders that will make your race day a positive and memorable event.

- Get yourself to the race with plenty of time for parking, walking to the start, and warming up with an easy jog.
- Set the countdown timer on your watch (if you have one) to beep every 10 minutes. When it goes off, drink electrolytes and check in with your running focuses, especially your posture and lean.
- Warm-up: Start warming up 20 minutes before the race—jog at least $1/2$ to 1 mile, depending on how much you feel your body needs. Do it at a very slow pace. Remember, you're just warming your muscles and getting your circulation moving. Light stretching after you've warmed up can sometimes alleviate pre-race jitters. Do your body looseners. They'll give you something focused to do that will keep your mind more in the present. Check your shoes one more time to make sure your shoelaces are comfortable and won't come untied (tuck in the loops). Jog for 10 minutes at an easy pace and then do some light stretches. After that, run a few light accelerations.
- Walk to where you plan to start and try to time it so you get there right before the gun goes off. You don't want to stand around letting your legs get stale. If you get there too early or the race has a late start, keep your legs moving. Shake them out, jog in place, walk around, do a few more strides.
- When the race starts, don't take off fast. Run easy for the first half-mile. When you're running for one hour or more, you don't need to worry about losing a couple of minutes up front, and it could make the difference between simply completing the distance (or maybe not) and having a great race.

- Check your pace after the first mile. If it's faster than your projected time, make an adjustment, relax, settle in. Don't say to yourself, "This pace doesn't feel that bad. I think I'll stay like this." You'll pay for it later. Check at the next mile marker to see if you've actually made the adjustment.
- Know beforehand approximately what time you want to be coming through your preset mile markers, and don't beat yourself up if you're behind a little—*caca pasa.*
- Drink *before* you're thirsty . . . take in electrolytes *before* you cramp . . . and adjust your form *before* you get tired.
- If you get tired, *always* do these three things:

    (1) Straighten your posture
    (2) Shorten your stride length
    (3) Lean from your ankles

    Additional, proven energy boosters: Look up, smile, talk to someone, take in your surroundings, find someone ahead of you and try to "reel" him or her in, swing your arms more, check in with your focuses, smile some more.
- Thank every race volunteer you see and cheer on every runner you pass.
- Race recovery: Cool down, stretch, do your leg drains, drink. When you get home, get into a hot bath ASAP.

    While you're sitting in your hot bath, think about what you just did. How do you feel about the day? Did you do what you set out to do? Did you exceed your expectations? Basically, do an end-of-run review, and *no matter what,* acknowledge to yourself the positives that came from the experience. If there is anything you would do differently, take it as a lesson learned and turn it into a focus for future training runs.

    Then massage your legs, drink more water, and eat a good solid protein meal. You deserve it!
- On the day after your race, ride your bike or walk to loosen up your legs. Stretch afterward and take another hot bath.

The success of your race will be directly proportional to the amount of planning and preparation that you put into it, on all levels. Some of these tips are to improve your physical advantage, and some are to improve your psychological advantage. Preparing yourself will help you to race your best and ace that test.

CHAPTER NINE

Getting the Most Chi from Your Food

The wisdom of life consists in the elimination of non-essentials.—LIN YU-TANG

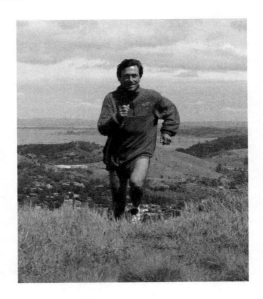

My belief is that your diet plays as important a role in your running as your training. That's a pretty bold statement, but I will also say that all of us could improve our running by improving our diet, and there is no way you will reach your potential in running without at some point addressing the issue of fueling. If your diet is high-octane and clean, you'll gain access to greater amounts of chi, which will provide the necessary fuel for higher levels of performance.

I don't know about you, but diet has never been an easy subject for me. The trouble probably started when I was a kid. With three other siblings, dinner was a free-for-all. No matter how many people sat down to eat, there always seemed to be only enough food for that number minus one. If I wanted a full meal, I had to dive in with everyone else, or I might be left with crumbs. Some of that early experience still has a hold on my eating behavior today; I can still eat like there's not going to be enough food. I've worked against that tendency since I first articulated it to myself over twenty-five years ago. I've gotten much better with it, but it still gets me sometimes. When I approach a meal in a relaxed and centered state, then I can slow down and enjoy the food, the company, and the experience. If I'm uptight, rushed, or just plain lazy, I can fall back into my former state quicker than a blink, and before I know it, I'm stuffed from overeating.

My issues with diet have, over the years, led me into the study and practice of getting the most from the food I eat. I've been blessed with some great teachers along the way. What I have found is that, as with ChiRunning, I need to set up the right conditions with my diet in order for chi to flow. This diet approach has worked well for me for twenty years and will provide you the guidelines for creating your own healthy diet. It's based on the accumulation of chi, which is really what eating should be all about. When your chi is flowing—whether from a good run or fresh, wholesome food—you get deeply nourished. Let's take a look at how to set up the right conditions.

PRINCIPLES OF CHIRUNNING APPLIED TO DIET

There is so much information, and even conflicting information, about diet out there that it's hard to know which advice will work best for you. What has helped me most has been keeping myself on a diet plan based on the ChiRunning principles. Now, you're probably thinking to yourself, "Yeah, right. Let's hear Diet Plan No. 10,005." But hear me out, because these are sensible guidelines that are helpful no matter what your current approach to diet is, whether you're a vegetarian or an omnivore. These principles each shed light on an aspect of diet in a wholesome way.

COTTON AND STEEL

Gather to your center and let go of all else. In other words, being mindful of your diet is the first step in learning to let go of the foods and eating habits that no longer serve your running or your health. If you want your diet to have a positive and long-lasting effect on your life, you must stay with your intentions and remember why you're doing it.

I love cheese. I could eat it every day, lots of it, but it wreaks havoc on my body. When I eat too much of it, my head gets stuffy, and I start to feel like a slug. So I limit myself to having cheese four times a week, because that's how much I can eat without my body feeling weird. As the principle says, Gather to your center (my knowledge that too much isn't good for me) and let go of all else (the other times during the week that I crave cheese). Stick to your plan—*that's* gathering to your center. And don't be drawn off track by all the things that will pull you off center and away from your plan. Anytime you gather to your center, you gather chi.

GRADUAL PROGRESS:
THE STEP-BY-STEP APPROACH

If you want to eat a cleaner, more wholesome diet—which I recommend—then allow yourself, and your body, some time to develop new habits with respect to food. Don't expect yourself to be great at your diet right away. It's not an easy subject to deal with, so take small but progressive steps to achieve your goals. Make small changes and let them be cumulative. It's just like learning the ChiRunning focuses— easier if you practice one at a time. When it's really in your system, you can add another brick to the foundation. Take your time and do it right. You'll build your chi by being solid within each step along the way.

For example, if you want to reduce your sugar intake (which I highly recommend as well), don't try to do it while you're also trying to cut back on caffeine and you have an intense project due at work in a few weeks. Just work on eliminating sugar, and when you're solid with that, begin to reduce your caffeine intake.

The amount of inner strength (chi) gained by improving one small aspect of your diet will give you the confidence to take on additional improvements. Rest assured that the cumulative effect of changing many aspects of your diet for the better will be transformative.

BALANCE

In order to maintain strong chi in your system, it is important to keep a balance among the nutrients necessary for your body to run well. My average seems to be 60 to 70% carbohydrates, 15 to 20% proteins, and 20 to 25% fats. You need to figure out what works for you. These are the three food groups that need to be in balance to fuel your body in the healthiest way. If your nutritional balance is out of whack, your available energy will fluctuate instead of being a nice steady burn. This will result in mood swings, peaks and valleys in your energy, and a certain level of unpredictability in your life in general.

It's not just that you need to be eating this proportional balance and your life will be better for it—it's also important that the carbohydrates, proteins, and fats are the highest quality. If you eat a high-quality diet, your body will be balanced in two ways: It will be nutritionally balanced with the right proportions of the three food groups, and it will also be balanced relative to the energy demands of an active life. High-quality foods = high-quality energy.

There are many things that will throw the body into a state of imbalance. Too many sweets, too much protein, and fried foods of any kind are a few examples. Our society seems driven by sweets and desserts. Sugar is in everything, especially processed foods, so it's easy to eat too many quick-burning sugars that send your blood sugar through the roof and then let you down with the subtlety of an auctioneer's gavel. The all-American diet also seems to contain some form of meat at least once a day; that's way more animal protein than your body needs. And our culture is hooked on saturated fats, which come mainly in the form of fried foods, processed cooking oils, butter, and animal products. A little bit is fine, but the amount that most people eat is out of balance with our bodies' real needs.

Another aspect of balance high on the list of anyone trying to regulate weight is between calories eaten and calories burned. If you want to lose weight, the balance has to swing toward burning more calories than you take in. If you'd like to gain weight, you'll need to eat more calories than you burn. It's a very simple formula that has ruled body proportions since the age of cavemen, and it's a great example of applied thermodynamics.

THE PYRAMID

The pyramid applies to your diet by suggesting that you have a very strong foundation in foods that deliver the most chi with the least amount of energy required to process them. As we go up the pyramid, we find foods that we still need in our diet, but in lesser amounts, and with the awareness that more of these foods is not better; they need to be consumed in proportion to the base of the pyramid.

This pyramid is not the official government-issued food pyramid. It's based on the diet I've been enjoying with great results for over twenty years. Once again, these are general guidelines. If you are a vegetarian or an endurance athlete, you'll modify this pyramid for your needs.

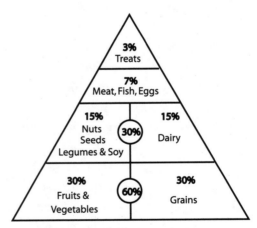

Figure 113—The Food Pyramid

Level 1: In order for you to have a healthy, clean-burning fuel supply, the foundation of your diet (the base of your pyramid) should be made up of grains, fruits, and vegetables. Not only are fruits and vegetables a good source of clean-burning carbohydrate fuel, they also provide your body with much-needed antioxidants, which are the free-radical scavengers. Free radicals in your cell tissues are produced by exercise and take much of the blame for everything from cancer to depletion of the immune system to premature aging. Whole grains are underappreciated and underutilized in our culture. They are slow-burning complex carbohydrates that provide a steady, long-term source of energy. When whole grains are processed and refined they become fast-burning, simple carbohydrates and low-octane fuel. My favorite whole grains are brown rice, kasha (buckwheat groats), oats, cornmeal, bulgur, and whole-wheat bread. Fully 60% of my diet comes from Level I of the pyramid—30% from fruits and vegetables and 30% from whole grains.

Level 2: The next level of foods makes up 30% of my diet: 15% from nuts, seeds, and legumes (soy products, nut butters, dried beans, and lentils) and 15% from dairy (cheese, yogurt, and milk). If you're not into dairy, you'll need to make up for your lack of fat and protein with plant-based products. But if you *are* into dairy, keep it to only 15% of your diet. You need Level 2 foods in your diet in order to maintain strong chi in your system, but the quantity (30%) is half the amount of Level 1.

Level 3: In my diet, the third level consists of meat, fish, and eggs, which I eat regularly but sparingly. It makes up a total of 7% of what I eat. I have fish once a week, meat once a week, and eggs one to two times a week. When animal protein is overconsumed, it depletes chi because of the intense processing it requires. When you do eat meat, it should be the highest quality possible, and organic, when available. If you're a vegetarian, you'll get protein from plant-based sources, such as legumes, and fats from oils, nuts, and nut butters.

Level 4: 3% of your diet should be from foods that are not necessarily eaten for nutritional reasons but are nourishing on other levels. I eat a yummy dessert once or twice a week, but when I'm tempted to eat too many sweets, I remind myself that I get more pleasure from having lots of chi than I do from being buzzed on sweets. There's no doubt about it, too much sugar depletes your immune system and can quickly throw a solid pyramid out of balance.

Caffeine falls into this group. Although it has been proven to enhance mental alertness and improve performance, it is also a diuretic that increases water loss. So, if you mix caffeine with running, take it with plenty of water.

The following foods are not doing you any favors nutritionally, and are not a part of the pyramid. The list includes such favorites as candy, condiments, processed foods, preservatives, additives, white flour (including bagels and most pastas), refined sugar, and sodas. These foods deplete your energy, and it's best to get them out of your diet altogether.

The pyramid serves as a visual reminder of where our strength really comes from, and shows the relative importance of certain types of foods in our lives.

NONIDENTIFICATION: GETTING YOURSELF OUT OF THE WAY

Nonidentification is really what maintaining a good diet is all about. We get stuck on ideas about ourselves and our diet that are not based on a true understanding of what our body needs. Anytime you're stuck on an idea about your weight or your diet, you're "identified," meaning you are using your ego and not your body to guide your decisions. Examples: "I'm addicted to chocolate." "I can't get going in the morning without my coffee." "I have to have meat every day, or I won't have the strength I need." "I need bread at lunch, or I'll still be hungry." Nonidentification with your diet means that in order to best support your current level of activity, you eat what you *need*, not what you *want*.

Nonidentification means you're acting totally in the best interests of your body. Imagine what it's like to be in a good place with your diet—to make strong, healthy decisions and be able to see them through.

The number one way to learn about your real needs is to Body

Sense. The proof of good diet is measured over time. How does your body feel immediately after eating, six hours later, the next day? Ask yourself and listen closely to your body's responses. It will tell you if you're on the right track or not.

Practical Steps for a Healthy Diet

One of the most profound things I have learned from studying healthy lifestyles is how important diet is in our lives. As I attempt to live more holistically, I am led to look at my diet in the same way I would any other activity—with a view to its part in the larger scheme of my life. I need to pay attention not only to *what* I eat but also *how much* I eat, *when* I eat, and *how* to eat.

WHAT TO EAT

If you want high-quality runs, *eat high-quality foods*. If your body isn't being supported by a good diet, it's like buying a Ferrari and putting low-octane gas in the tank. You can get much higher performance out of a car if it's running on premium fuel. It's as simple as that.

Whenever you sit down to a meal, think about where the food came from and whether you think it has a lot of life and energy still in it. There is no question that the most beautiful area of the grocery store is the produce section. There's a reason for that—the foods there have more life in them. Organic foods, including meat and dairy, are cleaner and closer to Nature than those that have been grown with chemical fertilizers and pesticides. I'm not going to give you specifics of what to eat (that's a whole 'nother book), but I do want you to start thinking about what you put in your mouth and why.

HIGH-CHI FOODS:

❑ Organic foods
❑ Fresh foods
❑ Freshly prepared foods
❑ Locally grown foods

LOW-CHI OR NO-CHI FOODS:

- ❏ Most canned foods
- ❏ Overcooked foods
- ❏ Processed and refined foods
- ❏ Fried foods
- ❏ Microwaved foods
- ❏ Foods with additives, preservatives, or coloring
- ❏ Pickled foods
- ❏ Condiments (commercially produced)
- ❏ Smoked foods

A great teacher set me up with my diet plan, and I am eternally grateful for having had this window into the power of a well-designed diet. Here's an overview.

I eat two main meals a day. I eat a hearty meal every morning. Three times a week it's a big bowl of hot whole-grain cereal loaded with nuts, seeds, and dried fruit. Once a week it's a substantial egg meal, and twice a week it's a grain and vegetable with nuts and sometimes cheese. Once a week I have a big bowl of yogurt with lots of nuts, seeds, raisins, and fruit. At midday I eat a light lunch, which might include dried fruit with nuts, or fresh fruit with cheese, or peanut butter with vegetable slices.

My weekly dinner menu looks something like this: a meat meal once a week, fish once a week, a huge salad once a week, and beans and rice once a week. On the three other nights I have grain-and-vegetable meals, sometimes with nuts, seeds, and/or cheese.

I always get the freshest organic ingredients available, and they are worth the extra cost. The meals are simple, delicious, and wonderfully satisfying.

WHEN TO EAT

Your body will work much better if your refueling is done in a cyclical manner: Eat your meals at the same times every day. This allows your stomach to work more efficiently, because the cycles of digestion are consistent in duration. Eating between meals makes your stomach work harder to digest freshly eaten food on top of food that is already in process—double duty. I eat my breakfast and dinner approximately twelve hours apart, because that's roughly the amount of time it takes for my stomach to completely digest a meal. I have a light lunch at midday, and if I need an energy boost during the late morning or afternoon, I'll have a cup of tea with honey (refined sugar spikes my blood sugar, and honey doesn't).

TIMING IS EVERYTHING

Not only is the quality of your food important, but, as they say, timing is everything. Your body will have different nutritional needs depending on your workout schedule. If you've just done a strenuous workout, one of your next two meals should be a solid protein meal to rebuild your muscles. It's also good to get in a hearty salad to put valuable minerals back into your system. By planning your meals ahead of time, you can match what is happening in your training schedule.

The basic rule of thumb is to eat a carbohydrate meal before a hard workout and a protein meal after. If you run in the morning, do your fueling the evening before. This allows you to get up, get dressed, and head out the door. A heavy meal the night before a hard workout might not be fully digested by the time you go out to run, which will slow you down considerably. High-octane, quick-burning fuel will help your workout to go much better.

If you eat before you run, be sure it's at least three hours prior. If you do have to eat before running, a banana helps your blood-sugar level and is a good source of potassium. Just don't eat a big meal before running or you might end up with heartburn, a stomachache, side stitches, or leaving it on the road somewhere. It's best to run on an empty stomach, even on race days. I've never heard of anyone starving to death on a run. In fact, if I'm hungry before I go running, it usually subsides within the first mile or two.

HOW TO EAT

To get the most chi out of your food, a few things will need to be in order. Your environment at mealtime has much to do with the quality of the chi you gain from the meal. At mealtime, you should settle down to take in nourishment and replenish your energy stores. The key to ensuring a high-quality meal is stillness.

Transitioning into a meal is the best way to get off to a nourishing start. First, make your eating environment a clear and settling space. Light a candle or decorate the eating area with a small flower arrangement. Remove any semblance of chaos. Make sure you have everything you need for your meal before you sit down so you don't have to get up once you've started eating.

Take a little time to remember what you're doing—you're taking in nourishment. As in your running, start off slowly. The beginning of the meal sets the pace for how it unfolds. If you start off too fast, the whole meal will be fast, and you'll finish with a full belly and still not feel nourished. Your food will not be well chewed, your stomach will have to work harder to digest it in its rough state, and you'll most likely feel like a toad when you get up from the table, instead of vibrant and replenished. Eat slowly and take small bites. (Do I sound like your mother yet?) Sit up straight and remember to breathe between bites.

Eating well and with a true respect for our bodies and the foods we eat is paramount to having a healthy body and maintaining a high-quality lifestyle.

RUNNING AND WEIGHT LOSS

Yes, you can lose weight through running, but here's the deal. Weight management is a product of calories in and calories out. The best way to regulate your weight is with a wise combination of diet *and* running. If you want to gain weight, eat more calories than you expend. If you want to lose weight, eat fewer calories than you expend. It's the law, and there is no naturally occurring way around it.

Don't let the job of maintaining a healthy weight fall solely on the shoulders of your running. One of the problems with that is when you can't run (because of injury, travel, etc.), you have nothing to fall back on to maintain your weight. My best advice is, If you want to regulate your weight, learn to regulate your diet first, and let your running regulate your toning.

Suggestions for a High-Chi Diet
- Eat two main meals a day with a light lunch between—breakfast is most crucial—and no snacks between meals.
- Eat about the same quantity for breakfast and dinner.
- Eat breakfast and dinner at about the same time every day.
- Generally, shoot for a balance of 15 to 25% fats, 60 to 70% carbohydrates, and 15 to 20% proteins.
- Not too many sweet treats or desserts (twice a week recommended).

These are only guidelines. Try them and see what works best for you. Every body is different.

CONCLUSION

Just as grains and vegetables are the foundation of a healthy diet, a good diet is the foundation for a successful running program and a vibrant life. I can't stress enough the importance of diet. The whole idea here is to put into your mouth only that which will deeply nourish you. Eating well *really* matters.

RECOMMENDED READING

These books on diet, nutrition, and natural health are some of the best and most thorough knowledge available, in my opinion.

Dynamic Nutrition for Maximum Performance, by Daniel Gastelu and Dr. Fred Hatfield, Avery Publishing Group, 1997.

The Encyclopedia of Natural Medicine (revised 2nd edition), by Michael Murray, N.D., and Joseph Pizzorno, N.D., Prima Publishing, 1998.

Smart Medicine for Healthier Living, by Janet Zand, L.Ac., O.M.D., Allan N. Spreen, M.D., C.N.C., James B. LaValle, R.Ph., N.D., Avery Publishing Group, 1999.

Between Heaven and Earth: A Guide to Chinese Medicine, by Harriet Beinfield, L.Ac., and Efrem Korngold, L.Ac., O.M.D., Ballantine Books, 1991.

Feeding the Whole Family, by Cynthia Lair, Moon Smile Press, 1997.

CHAPTER TEN

Run as You Live, Live as You Run

There is a life-force within your soul, seek that life.
There is a gem in the mountain of your body, seek that mine.
O traveler, if you are in search of That
Don't look outside, look inside yourself and seek That.—RUMI

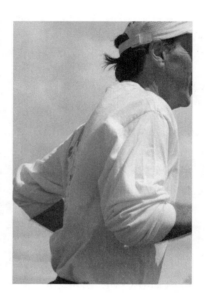

just got back from my Sunday-cruise run, and I feel like a new person. My week was way busier than normal, and I needed to get out of the house and into the hills. I arrived at the trailhead feeling a bit groggy from working on the book until all hours the night before, and I was really looking forward to the run because I *knew* I would return to my car feeling better than when I left. Indeed, I was able to totally turn my energy around within two hours. In the past, it might have taken days or weeks. There are a few personal activities I have to thank for that: a consistent running program, a high-quality diet, good clean communication with those close to me, and a keen awareness that letting up on any one of the above is not an option.

I live in a very small, close-knit neighborhood with neighbors who'll knock on your door and tell you your car windows are down when it starts to rain. Marge lives across the street. We consider her the village elder, because she cares so much about all the families up and down the block. She's been here since just after World War II, back when houses sold for five figures. What I most appreciate about her is her attitude toward life. When I see her out in her garden watering the plants, I usually ask how she's doing, to which she inevitably replies, with a twinkle in her eye, "I've got a lot to be thankful for . . . I woke up today. And when you get to be my age, things like that are important." I couldn't agree more on both counts. She is a model for me of someone who takes advantage of every day, because she knows she might not be around tomorrow. She's fit as a fiddle and sharp as a tack because she has spent years eating well, exercising, caring for others, and generally holding the attitude that life is something to be treasured . . . every day.

Our culture offers little in terms of training us how to live and appreciate life from the inside out. So much of our focus is on the external that little attention is put on considering what goes on internally. I'm not suggesting we should all be isolationists or self-centered. I'm saying we can all best contribute to society if we first and foremost sense and acknowledge our own feelings, then act from a sense of who we really are, not from an idea of what will earn us the most positive or avoid the most negative responses.

How does one get to this elusive place of centeredness? Of all the principles discussed in Chapter 2, the most important is Cotton and Steel. Whenever you go out for a run, practice this principle, and it will guide you to be centered in your running and in your life. Cotton and Steel is infused within all the ChiRunning themes—planning, staying relaxed, breathing, working with balance in mind, taking small steps to ensure gradual progress, practicing nonidentification in the face of challenges and setbacks, and building a strong base that is unshakable in its support for your actions. By consistently using these themes in your ChiRunning program, you'll begin to see how they apply in your life.

I have a client who tells me that whenever she comes up against a situation in which she feels at a loss, she asks herself, "If this were a run, how would I approach the solution, and what adjustment would I make?" She says it never fails to help her find the answer inside her own body of knowledge. Here's a letter she sent recently:

> Danny,
>
> I think the real benefit of ChiRunning is not only being able to run without pain but applying the ideas to all aspects of my life. I am now working on trying to use the "form" to help me live my life more freely and easily, free from stress and other types of pain (e.g., emotional, intellectual). I am seeing that the same principles that are used to make running less of an effort and more efficient can be used to help my life be more calm and peaceful in a world that seems crazy and chaotic at times. If I can try to relax when I feel tired or overwhelmed, or if I return to my center when I feel stress or anxiety, then I will have truly adopted the principles of ChiRunning. From a purely physical viewpoint, ChiRunning can be used to run faster and farther and will definitely make me a better and more relaxed runner. However, I feel that there is so much more to it than that. By practicing the principles of Body Sensing and efficiently using my muscle energy to enjoy my runs, it teaches me that I can learn to sense myself physically and emotionally in all situations and to not waste energy as I journey through life. I know that incorporating this philosophy with a holistic focus will enable me to achieve a true sense of peace and happiness. *Aga Goodsell*

For me, the practice of ChiRunning helps maintain a clear, strong sense of connection with my body—which translates, in no uncertain terms, to inner freedom. The freedom to not be intimidated by challenges I face. The freedom to follow my intuition instead of second-guessing my choices. The freedom to allow my present condition to guide my future but not rule it.

This sense of freedom is what makes it possible to live life creatively. My wife always tells me that she doesn't consider herself a creative person. She compares herself to the artists and creative people she has surrounded herself with her entire life, but she doesn't feel she's in their league. Quite the contrary, I see her as being highly creative, not only in how she lives her life but in being who she is. She is rock-solid in her beliefs and holds to them, knowing they are based in Truth. She creates her own life every day by embodying her beliefs and knowledge of what's best. She's not driven by the goals of others, and I rarely see her going along with the general trends of our culture without deeply questioning their benefits and drawbacks. She holds to her center and meets her challenges with the grace of a T'ai Chi master. And she is taking the utmost care in creatively passing on that knowledge to our daughter.

Creativity has many forms, and it's my assertion that we can all be creative beings if we can learn to center our lives with programs that allow us to experience ourselves being grounded in our bodies. Embodying the Cotton and Steel principle allows you to be driven by what is inside of you, not by what is inside of someone else.

T'ai Chi is based on the principle of Cotton and Steel, which means moving and living from one's center. It's a theme that we could all use in our approach to this fast-paced world. Things might not always fall exactly how you'd like them to. But when you're centered, you can be creative and fluid in responding to anything that happens.

Master Xu says that whenever he fights an opponent in training, he has no idea what is going to happen, because it's a creative act. He told me about an incident that happened just after he moved to this country from China. He was walking home from the grocery store when a gang of six guys (some with knives) surrounded him on the street and demanded money. When he refused to give it to them, they came in for the attack. BIG mistake. The next thing he remembers is that all of them were lying on the ground around him; one had to be taken to the hospital. He said his body just took over and responded in an instant to everything that was coming at him. There was no thought process involved; it was a purely creative act. I experience a similar type of creativity when I'm running down a single-track trail at high speed. I get into an inner zone of stillness while rocks and trees come at me in a blur of motion. I watch my body do the running while I sit back and enjoy the ride. That's when running feels more like dancing than danger.

How to turn what you learn from ChiRunning into useful everyday habits would fill a book by itself (which might happen). The easiest way to transfer all of this information to your life in general is to go back and read this book from the start, and every time you see the words "run" and "running," just substitute "live" and "living." Watch how they work interchangeably.

GUIDELINES FOR CHILIVING

Use the Chi-Skills from Chapter 3 when approaching everything from a business project to grocery shopping. Practice them all the time. The best way to begin transferring your ChiRunning knowledge into the rest of your life is to start each day with the Body Sensing exercise from Chapter 3. Do it consistently, every day if possible. Use it to get in touch with your body first thing in the morning. Believe me, it's better for you than a cup of coffee: It launches you into the morning conscious of your body instead of your head. Later in the day, when you're sitting in your car or at your desk, return to Body Sensing and review your body scan. If you sense any tension or discomfort, you can soften that area and move on. Do little remembrances like this all day long—sensing and correcting, making adjustments as you go. When your posture isn't straight, make an adjustment. When you find yourself not breathing, make an adjustment. If you find yourself holding tension somewhere, relax it. If you want to build a center, practice bringing your attention to the spine all day long.

Make your workday a moving meditation in which you constantly bring attention to your spine. Focusing on spine and breath are two centering devices that have been used in meditation practices for centuries. Sitting in meditation, one focuses on keeping the spine still, which then positions movement as its complement. In this way one learns to accommodate stillness in the midst of activity. Remembering your spine and your breath brings you into the present moment, from which many possibilities of action can spring forth.

When you're running, keeping your posture in line brings you to your center. When you're *not* running, the same thing applies.

Opening New Doors

A little over three years ago, Eddie started running. He had grown up in Manhattan, and the only time he ever ran was when he was late for the A train. His brother needed a kidney transplant, so Eddie took up running to get himself into the physical shape needed to be a healthy donor. He never ended up having to donate his kidney, thankfully, but it got him started. He subsequently moved to California and ran more often and, within a year, found himself running his first marathon. The second year, after taking a series of ChiRunning classes, he ran five marathons; this past year he ran eight marathons, three 50Ks (31.1 miles), a fifty-miler, and a 100K (62 miles!). If he keeps it up at this rate, I figure he should be able to run to Hawaii sometime next year.

What makes Eddie's story remarkable is that he is 56 years old. More than anything, it has been his attitude that has allowed him to run these distances without being intimidated by them.

He has practiced the focuses since his first ChiRunning class two years ago, and they are now a great set of tools that he uses in every run. Now, whenever he meets a challenging section of a run, he knows there is always something he can do to help himself through. When I asked him what goes through his head when he considers running longer and longer distances, he told me that all he had to do was the required preparation—which for him meant consistent training and enjoyment of the process.

He has an incredibly infectious positive attitude, which I believe frees him to do what he needs to do without wasting energy worrying about how it's going to get done or what the outcome will be. When I asked him to sum up his attitude about running, he said, "Any day that you don't finish a run is still a day that you went out for a beautiful run. If that's the downside, then there's no downside!"

ChiRunning leaves you with a sense of confidence that if you approach anything with a realistic vision, a well-thought-out plan, and a consistent, step-by-step approach, you can accomplish great things.

It's about doing the necessary work of maintaining and carefully building your base so that growth—albeit slow sometimes—is always in a forward direction. When you feel centered in yourself, with the confidence that years of mindful living produce, you are freed up to live your life creatively while keeping to your practice. You are externally consistent with the actions that allow you to live a rich life while staying internally free. It's all about enjoying the process of growth and not being overfocused on results.

As you become increasingly familiar with the Chi-Skills, you will begin to open windows and doors to levels that you never dreamed possible. Seeing each level and finding new sets of possibilities there is like taking the elevator up in a skyscraper and checking out the view every ten stories. Each new vista is quite different. What seemed larger than life from the ground floor looks much smaller and less significant when you are looking down at it from the upper stories. When you get to the top of the building, you notice that the city is really surrounded by miles of open space and places to explore.

Creative running, or creative living, means developing your skills to the point where you're not intimidated by anything thrown at you. As the ChiRunning skills become more integrated into your regular routine, living an extraordinary life will seem normal.

Appendix
A Guide to the Muscles Referred to in the Book

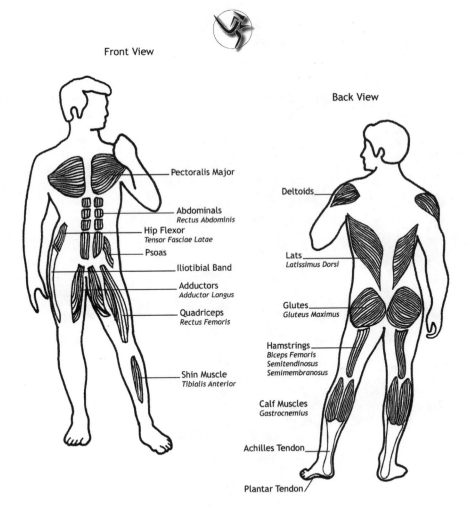

Front View

Back View

Pectoralis Major

Deltoids

Abdominals
Rectus Abdominis
Hip Flexor
Tensor Fasciae Latae
Psoas

Iliotibial Band

Adductors
Adductor Longus

Quadriceps
Rectus Femoris

Shin Muscle
Tibialis Anterior

Lats
Latissimus Dorsi

Glutes
Gluteus Maximus

Hamstrings
Biceps Femoris
Semitendinosus
Semimembranosus

Calf Muscles
Gastrocnemius

Achilles Tendon

Plantar Tendon

Index

About the Authors

Danny Dreyer, creator of the ChiRunning technique, an esteemed running coach and a nationally ranked ultramarathon runner, has over thirty years of running experience, and is a student of internationally renowned T'ai Chi Master George Xu. He has been published in *Runner's World* and *Running Times,* and is the author of his own monthly ChiRunning newsletter. Danny has taught the ChiRunning method to thousands of people with profound results. Danny lives a lifestyle steeped in holistic living, meditation, and personal wellness. He lives in the San Francisco Bay area with his wife, Katherine, and daughter, Journey.

Katherine Dreyer combines over twenty years of experience publishing information about health and fitness, with sixteen years of study of Eastern philosophy and practices. She was president of New Hope Communications, the leading communications company for the natural health business and vice president of HealthShop.com. Katherine works with Danny to develop ChiRunning, ChiLiving, and ChiWalking.

CHIRUNNING FOR SWIMMERS

Many runners, especially triathletes, ask me if there is a way to apply all of the ChiRunning focuses to swimming. And, without reservation, I send them to the Total Immersion swimming program developed by master coach and Masters distance swimmer Terry Laughlin. For years, Terry's approach to efficient swimming has proven to be the technique of choice for swimmers of all levels and distances, but particularly for novices and "struggling swimmers." His revolutionary method, which he calls "Fish-like Swimming," replaces the traditional focus on pulling, kicking, and swimming longer/harder with a focus on being balanced, "slippery," and fluent. Using the same core principles for swimming that ChiRunning uses for running, he teaches a mindful, centered approach that any swimmer can learn. There will never be a ChiSwimming. With Total Immersion swimming there doesn't need to be. If you're pleased with the effect ChiRunning has had on your running, you owe it to yourself to check out Total Immersion swimming. An update of his bestselling book, *Total Immersion,* will be released in 2004. www.totalimmersion.net